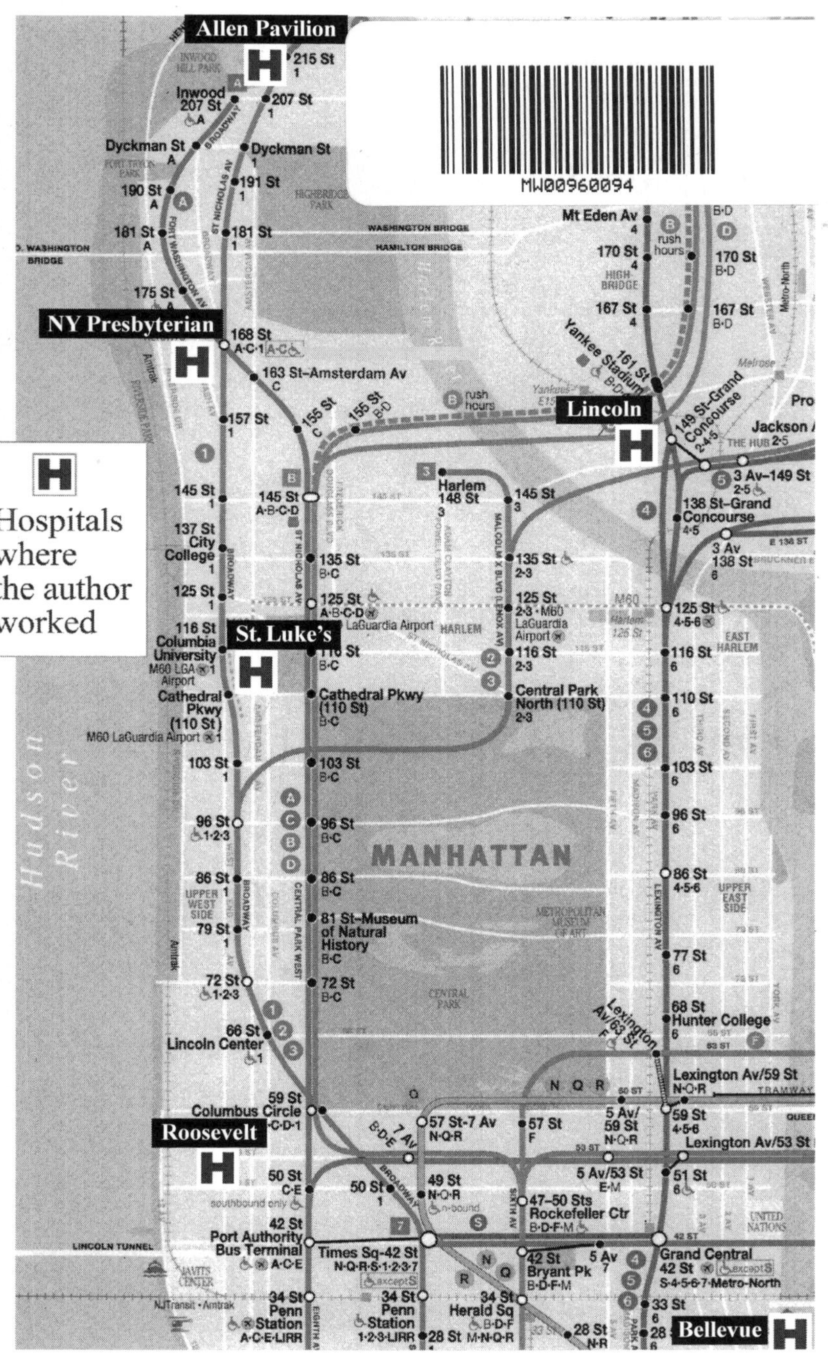

NYC Subway Map © Metropolitan Transportation Authority. Used with permission.

Praise for

Laboring:
Stories of a New York City Hospital Midwife

"This book brings 'Call the Midwife' into modern, urban medicine. Well written and concise, you'll be transported to the joy, fear and angst of the maternity ward of a busy hospital. A must read for anyone who celebrates the miracle of life."

Hon. Nancy Dusek-Gomez, retired Justice, Massachusetts' Trial Court

"***Laboring*** gives voice to the dedicated, unassuming, and often silenced work of the midwife. Riveting, engaging, emotional, and present, this book transports the reader into the literal hands-on world of a New York City hospital midwife as she encounters the demanding life and death responsibilities of being with woman."

Amínata Maraesa PhD, Anthropology Department, Hunter College

"Share in the joys, excitement and sorrows of a midwife practicing in inner city hospitals. The author vividly captures the extraordinary empathy that midwives bring to women. Be transported into the shoes of a midwife as she confronts the challenges and satisfactions of providing high quality care to some of the city's lowest income and needy families."

Frances T. Thacher, CNM, MSN. FACNM

"I was so taken with this book that I read it in one day. It should be read by a wide audience. It really shows the heart of being a midwife."

Karen Burgin, LM, Editor *Metro Midwives*

"***Laboring*** is the real life inspiring story of a midwife in New York City who copes with the challenges of working in environments where the talents, skills and intuition of midwives are often undervalued by hospital hierarchy and where her patients at times struggle with the effects of poverty, HIV infection, substance abuse, mental illness as well as other disabilities. This is a beautiful, compelling and at times heart wrenching book that will strike a chord with anyone who works in the field of childbirth as well as all of us who have been transformed by birth and parenthood."

Margot Hodes, Ed.D., M.A., Adjunct Assistant Professor of Health Education, Columbia University, Teachers College, Childbirth Educator, Certified Lactation Counselor

Laboring

Stories of a New York City Hospital Midwife

By Ellen Cohen

Cohen, Ellen 1st ed. p. cm.
Stories of a New York City Hospital Midwife / Ellen Cohen

ISBN-13: 978-1492803997
ISBN-10: 1492803995
Library of Congress Control Number: 2013920034

Laboring: Stories of a New York City Hospital Midwife

number of pages 172

Contact information:
cnmellen48@gmail.com

For my children, grandchildren and patients.

And for midwives everywhere.

Acknowledgements

Thanks go to many people who helped make this book a reality. My husband John and sister Naomi midwifed this project from vague thoughts to an actual book with their continuous encouragement, reading and re-reading the evolving manuscript and technical support.

Writing teachers Kelly Caldwell and Cullen Thomas always pushed me to go deeper. Poet Veronica Golos contributed insightful editing, probing questions and the title. Lallan Schoenstein designed the book and its cover. Marta Szabo shared her expertise.

Many people read various versions of the manuscript but these seven helped to improve it by their criticisms and suggestions: Karen Burgin, Bernard Catalinotto, Dalia Griñan, Sandy Kohler, Donna Lazarus, Frances Thacher and Diane Tose.

Bridget Bartolini invited me to read "Housekeepers" at the Bronx Museum to an audience similar to my patients. The positive response I received there was an important validation that my writing could reach out beyond the usual midwife-friendly circles.

Several colleagues are mentioned by name as those who taught, mentored and worked alongside me. It was not possible to include all the wonderful midwives whose paths crossed mine over the years, but I want to thank my teachers at the State University of New York Downstate midwifery program 1982-1983 in Brooklyn: Evelyn Brown, Betty Carrington, Phyllis Gorman, Lily Hsia and Mazel Lindo. And no discussion of maternal-infant health in New York City would be complete without the name of Dorothea Lang, longtime Director of the Nurse-Midwifery Program at this city's Maternity, Infant Care and Family Planning Projects. Her vision and lifelong dedication to our profession were vital in bringing midwifery care to huge numbers of poor and underserved women. Dorothea also hired me for my first job as a midwife.

Finally, thanks to all the colleagues, co-workers, comrades and comadres who taught me what it means to be a working woman.

CONTENTS

Foreword

There is a long list of begats in Genesis, Chapter 11, naming the fathers, but not the mothers who bore all the generations of sons and daughters. After decades caring for women as a midwife in New York City hospitals I want to tell the mothers' stories. I also hope to explain the midwifery approach to maternity care.

Aside from the first few months at Bellevue and notes taken on the bus rides through the Bronx I did not keep a journal of my student years or professional life as either a nurse or midwife. It seemed too time-consuming and self-absorbed. Besides, what use could it possibly be?

So almost everything in this book comes from memory – with its searing impressions and deep gaps; the clarity of hindsight and the fog of forgetting. The writing is as true as these imperfect tools can make it.

Many of the vignettes may seem truncated or incomplete. That was often the nature of my work: intense but brief interactions with a woman who I never met before and who I might never see after delivering her baby. Not an ideal way to practice midwifery, but I tried to bring dignity and grace to those encounters, knowing that a mother always remembers the births of her children. Or I might form a relationship with a patient over many months of prenatal care but not be on duty when she delivered.

Names and certain details about patients have been changed to preserve their privacy. Co-workers' real names are used in many instances (when remembered). Any person whose story might cause pain or embarrassment is not referred to by his or her actual name.

Basic facts about pregnancy and birth must be included so that readers can understand what is happening in several stories. More detailed medical information can be found in the Notes to the Reader section at the end of the book for those who are interested.

Some of the practices described in the stories have been modified or discarded over time and do not reflect current knowledge or practice. Good riddance to strapping women's hands and feet to the delivery table, routine episiotomies, shaving off pubic hair, rushing to cut the umbilical cord and snatching newborn from mother so that hospital routines can be carried out! But I could not change the accounts of how I practiced twenty or thirty years ago without doing grievous harm to the truth.

Here are the mothers' stories, as well as mine. They are meant to illuminate the pain, joy and occasional heartbreak of childbirth, as well as shed light on the challenges facing both mothers and midwives.

Chapter 1

Mia

"I'm not pregnant so nobody's going to examine me. Get your hands away from my pussy." Pause. "No, I don't use drugs." Pause. "Just my Thorazine and my crack… And I'm not taking the Thorazine now anyhow." Thorazine is an anti-psychotic medication prescribed for people suffering from schizophrenia.

The woman's loud voice came from the Labor and Delivery triage room where patients were evaluated to determine whether they were in labor or had a complication of pregnancy and should be admitted or could be sent home.

Peeking into the room I saw the patient crawling on the floor, naked. Her belly was term pregnancy size; amniotic fluid trickled down her thighs. The doctor, a third-year resident, was also pregnant, in her seventh month, and obviously unclear as to how to proceed. Nothing in her training had prepared her for a situation quite like this.

I sympathized with the pregnant resident. Perhaps fearful for her own physical safety, she was uncertain how to care for such a resistant patient and feeling the general anxiety that psychotic people arouse with their irrational behavior.

Entering the room I leaned down and addressed the patient on the floor.

"Hi, my name is Ellen." No need to mention that I am a midwife. If she was familiar with that term it would only provoke more resistance to the suggestion that she was pregnant. I let my white coat and stethoscope offer my general credentials as some kind of medical person.

"How are you feeling?" I asked.

"Terrible," she replied. "I have a terrible stomach ache and my bowels are in an uproar." She stood up to show me her aching stomach.

"Let me put you in a nice clean bed and check what's hurting you," I offered. Grabbing a hospital gown from the linen cart, I helped her slip into it and made a bow with the ties that held it closed over her swollen abdomen. She did not object.

"We'll be in Room 4," I told the doctor, picking up the blank triage form and the papers that Emergency Medical Services left when they brought the patient here by ambulance from a mid-Manhattan subway station. The resident did not resist my taking charge.

"What's your name?" I asked the patient.

"Mia," she answered. We walked out of the triage area and down the hall to a room in Labor and Delivery. "Here comes another one of these terrible pains," she alerted me. I rubbed her lower back until the pain passed. Then Mia climbed into the bed. I covered her with a sheet. Beatrice, a very capable, very proper British nurse, was assigned to this admission. Sounding like she was inviting her to tea with the queen, Beatrice requested Mia's permission to take her vital signs. Mia lifted her pink tongue for the thermometer and held out her arm for the blood pressure cuff. When this was done and another pain had come and gone it was my turn.

"Mia, can I listen to your heart and lungs and feel your stomach?" I asked. She nodded yes. Her heart and lung sounds were normal. From her pubic bone to the top of her abdomen I measured 36 centimeters with a paper tape. This is a normal size for a fetus at term and I estimated that the baby weighed about 6 ½ pounds. My fingers told me that the baby was in the head first or vertex position, ready for an uncomplicated birth. On the left her abdomen felt smooth, which indicated that the baby's back was nestled on that side. With my stethoscope a little below and to the left of Mia's navel I heard the baby's heart beating strongly, about 144 times a minute. On the right were moving bumps – the baby's hands, feet, elbows or knees. All that activity was another sign of a healthy baby.

With the next pain Mia squirmed away from me. I saw the uterine muscle tighten, her face contort, and didn't need any high tech equipment, or even my fingers, to know the contractions were strong.

I asked the standard health history questions. Mia denied having any illnesses, told me she gave birth to a daughter three years ago. There were no problems with that pregnancy or birth. The little girl lived with an aunt, she said.

Now I had enough data about this pregnancy to know how to safely care for mother and baby. Mia's temperature, pulse and blood pressure were fine. The baby's heartbeat was strong. There was one fetus in the right position for a normal birth. My patient did not remember her last menstrual period but the size of her belly indicated a full term baby. The bag of water surrounding the baby had broken. The amniotic fluid contained no meconium, the tarry stool that can indicate fetal distress, nor flecks of vernix, the cheesy substance that protects the fetus' skin and is more likely to be present in a premature birth. The fluid was clear and without any odor to make me suspect infection.

Women in advanced labor often are agitated. Except for denying being pregnant, Mia's behavior was not that unusual for a woman almost ready to enter the pushing stage of birth.

With the patient settled in bed I left her momentarily with Beatrice and went to the nurses' station to give a full report on Mia's status to the rest of the staff.

"What's going on here?" the attending physician in charge of Labor and Delivery demanded.

Using obstetric jargon I summarized the information about Mia's labor, adding, "The patient apparently has a history of schizophrenia treated with Thorazine, but is currently not taking any medication and admits to using crack cocaine. She denies being pregnant and refuses any vaginal examination. The pediatricians have been notified and we requested a psychiatric consult."

"She must deliver in a delivery room with pediatrics present," he ordered.

"A pediatrician will be here, but going to the delivery room is impossible," I told him. He stalked away without arguing. Later I learned that he had told the young resident to have Mia sign out "against medical advice" – in effect, send the patient out into the street to give birth – when she refused a vaginal examination.

Returning to Room 4 I found Mia thrashing around in bed, the sheets in a tangled pile at her feet. Her rectum bulged out under the pressure of the baby's head. Having attended thousands of women in labor I knew this was a sign that her cervix, the opening of the womb, was now fully dilated.

"Push, Mia, push," I encouraged her. "Everything will come out and you will feel much better."

Beatrice started setting up the room for the birth. She turned on the warmer for the baby bassinet and opened a pack with sterile cord clamps, scissors, gauze and iodine cleansing solution. I put on cap, mask, gown and sterile gloves.

Stool was coming out of Mia's rectum under the pressure of the baby's advancing head and she was reaching down between her legs and smearing feces over herself and the bed with her hands. I kept cleaning her off with gauze pads, discarding the dirty gloves and putting on new sterile pairs. Soon we could see a tiny patch of the baby's soft black curls. The pediatrician waited right outside the labor room door. All the equipment for resuscitating a baby was ready just in case.

With each contraction a little more of the baby's head became visible. Between contractions Beatrice listened to the fetal heart with her stethoscope, the bell pressed low on Mia's abdomen. The nurse tapped out the beat with the raised forefinger of her free hand. The baby's pulse was normal. With a few more pushes it would be born.

Mothers feel intense pressure from the baby's head and a burning sensation in the perineum during these moments just before birth. Mia must have been feeling that; she jumped over the raised side rails and out of bed, as if that would help her escape the pain, and ran out of the room into the large open area near the nurses' station. After a split second of shocked disbelief Beatrice and I ran right behind her. Mia leaned against the wall with the next contraction as the baby's head emerged.

"Squat down, Mia," I told her. She flopped to the floor on her back, refusing to open her legs and batting away my hands as I knelt beside her attempting to help ease out the baby's shoulders. Beatrice was trying to stop Mia from hitting me. The baby was wriggling its way into the world. I sensed a semi-circle of spectators behind us, their eyes riveted on the drama being played out on the floor.

The baby delivered himself and cried lustily. Somebody handed me the cord clamps and scissors and patted me encouragingly on the back. I cut the umbilical cord and announced "Boy!"

"It IS a baby," Mia said as she propped herself up on one elbow to see the pediatrician take her son from my hands and into a warm towel. "But I'm always losing things…I don't think I should keep him," she added with a startling clarity that broke my heart.

"The afterbirth needs to come out now," I said, getting to my feet and helping her off the floor, escorting her back to the labor room and into bed. "It's soft and mushy, like a thick pancake, and doesn't hurt. Just push once more with the next pain." A few minutes later the placenta delivered. I rubbed her abdomen to help the uterus contract and avoid bleeding. Beatrice got Mia's permission to give her an injection of Pitocin, a drug used to prevent postpartum hemorrhage, but the patient adamantly refused to let me check her vagina for lacerations. There was no bleeding to indicate any such problem, so I was not concerned. Careful inspection of the placenta's liver-like lobes assured me that it was intact and complete: nothing was left inside the uterus to cause infection or hemorrhage.

"How do you feel now?" I asked, untying the surgical mask from my sweaty face, pulling off the blue operating room cap and snapping off the now very unsterile gloves.

"Hungry!" she said.

Mia took a shower and enjoyed two lunch trays. The pool of blood and amniotic fluid on the floor where she gave birth was mopped up. Normal routines were reestablished. The drama was over, although I imagined gossip about this birth was only beginning. I sat at a desk in the nurses' station, just finished filling out the medical record and birth certificate, when the psychiatrist arrived on Labor and Delivery. We had paged him nearly two hours earlier to consult about an out-of-control patient in our unit.

"Who is taking care of the psych patient?" he asked. The ward clerk and nurses all pointed to me.

"Dr. Richards," he introduced himself. "Are you the OB attending?" I was in my late 40s and in the hospital hierarchy people sometimes confuse older age with higher rank.

"I'm the midwife," I answered.

"But who is the physician responsible for this patient?" he wanted to know, "I need to speak to him."

Wrong title, wrong pronoun. His insult opened the floodgate of emotions that this birth triggered in me.

"When she was crawling on the floor saying she was not pregnant, I took care of her," I said. "When she was smearing her feces everywhere, I took care of her." My normally soft voice was rising. The psychiatrist cringed away from me but the wall at his back prevented him from retreating far. "When she delivered her baby running down the hall, I took care of her. You want to know about her? Ask me!" My heart was pounding. Dr. Richards' face turned red. He mumbled a lame excuse about needing to know her vital signs.

"Then look at the nurses' notes in the chart," I said, pointing to the just-completed paperwork, and escaped to the female locker room.

There I could be alone to cry. I wept for the tragedy of Mia and her baby, for all the Mia's and all their children. I cried for the life experience that had prepared me for precisely this moment: my own son had been diagnosed with schizophrenia ten years earlier and was lost in the dark pit of that disease. My heart holds a special place for people suffering from mental illness. Mia's irrational behavior did not frighten or unnerve me. I felt no need to insist on the reality that she was pregnant if her perception was that she had a stomach ache.

When my tears were exhausted I thanked all the midwives whose accumulated wisdom enabled me to safely deliver this woman without tying her down like an animal or assaulting her with a forced pelvic exam. I thanked my wise midwife professor, Lily Hsia, who taught me, "Always ask the patient. Ask her what **she** thinks is the problem." That was the key that unlocked the door to caring for Mia. Her stomach hurt. I listened to her complaint and treated that pain.

Mia was sent to the psychiatric unit rather than to the post-partum floor with the other mothers. I visited her two days after the birth. Her milk had come in, making her breasts hard and painful. I filled latex examination gloves with ice, put these cold "hands" on her swollen breasts and wrote an order in her chart for ice packs every four hours.

About a week later, dutifully taking her Thorazine and obeying the rules, Mia earned a pass to go outside and smoke a cigarette. She never came back; in hospital speak she "absconded."

The aunt who was caring for Mia's older child, bless her, also took the baby boy.

* * *

Shortly before this birth, I had been offered a position at a clinic for HIV-infected women and children. I drew two columns on a sheet of lined notebook paper, listing the pros of the possible change in one column and the cons in the other. Weighing them objectively still left me undecided. Perhaps rather than seeking a purely rational reason for taking this job or refusing it I was looking for a "sign," an emotional reaction that would help me make up my mind. The birth of Mia's baby provided that. Something in me changed after delivering her. I felt unafraid to confront new challenges and accepted the job.

CHAPTER 2

What is a midwife?

When people hear that I am a midwife they usually respond with one of these comments:

"That means you do home births, right?" or

"What a happy profession" or

"Midwives are great. A midwife delivered … both my children … my grandson … my sister's baby" or

"Is that like a doula?" or

"What is a midwife?"

Home births?

Many people are surprised to learn that more than 95 percent of midwife deliveries in this country take place in hospitals. The public associates midwives with home births because of the media attention to that part of our practice. The popular BBC series, "Call the Midwife," is set in 1950s London, where midwives pedal their bicycles to deliver patients at home. Chris Bohjalian's best-seller *Midwives* and the Ricki Lake/Abby Epstein documentary, "The Business of Being Born," both feature home birth midwives caring for women who are well educated about childbirth and choose to deliver at home.

My patients did not always have homes. They were randomly assigned to me in busy clinics and no-frills hospital labor rooms where it was often a struggle to give each woman the time and attention she deserved. They were among the more than 40 percent of pregnant women in the U.S. whose low-wage jobs, unemployment or lack of health benefits make them eligible for Medicaid-type insurance for maternity and newborn care. [See Notes to the Reader.]

A Happy Profession

Yes, midwifery is a happy profession – most of the time. It can be addictive with the adrenalin of being a key actor at one of life's peak moments: the natural miracle of birth. Terrible when things go badly. Filled with sleepless nights and overwhelming guilt when something goes wrong, whether we are responsible or not. Potentially dangerous from the constant exposure to blood and the possibility of becoming infected with hepatitis or HIV. Intensely physical in the way we touch our patients, stand for hours, bend and push, work through the night, listen to the faint tapping of a fetal heartbeat through a stethoscope on a mother's belly, sniff for the smell of amniotic fluid, use our fingertips to measure and probe, our hands and voices to comfort.

Our knowledge of women's bodies is deeper than a lover's. We know the bubblegum pink of the cervix and how it lies purplish and flaccid after birth; the liver red of a placenta; the toughness of a caul, those translucent membranes forming the bubble in which the fetus floats. We feel the gelatinous texture of the umbilical cord as, with a snip of scissors, we irrevocably separate mother and newborn.

The happy part for me is not so much the babies. Babies are precious, adorable. I love their fleshy newborn smell, the silkiness of their skin, the fine hair, the way their tiny fingers curl around the bigger finger of an adult. I love to watch their little lips rooting for a mother's nipple and the whole-body shiver of satisfaction as they latch on and begin to suck. .

But for me the best part is working with women from all over the world, from different cultures, speaking different languages.

Pregnancy can be a time of infinite possibilities. A woman may do things for the baby she carries that she could not do for herself, end bad habits or patterns, reach higher to be her best self. When a baby is born so is a new mother. The gift I want to give her is awareness of her own strength and capabilities.

My Midwife

When people have been cared for by a midwife I love to hear their stories. Sometimes I know the midwife they are talking about. There are about 250 of us in New York City and I have worked, taught, or attended meetings with many of them.

"Midwives give such personal care," a woman, now a grandmother, recently told me, remembering the relationship more than 30 years ago. "I had complications and needed a Cesarean section," she said. "The doctors at Harlem hospital saved my life, and my baby's." But the person she still calls "my midwife" and whose name she will never forget is the one who cared for her during the pregnancy, and was my colleague for many years, the wonderful Gloria Dawan. For decades Ms. Dawan was one of the only Muslim midwives practicing in a New York City hospital. She was revered in that community and women traveled from all over to be cared for by her. Administrators at the hospital where Ms. Dawan worked apparently never realized her fame and how many patients she attracted.

Like a doula?

Doulas have gotten lots of publicity recently. They accompany a woman during labor, providing emotional support and physical comfort measures. They have no medical role or responsibilities, but studies show that the presence of such a person increases the chances of a normal birth, decreases the need for pain medication and enhances the mother's feeling of satisfaction with her experience.

What is a midwife?

Our specialty is normal pregnancy and birth. We focus on each patient as a whole human being, and birth as a psychosocial, as well as biological, event. Now educated at a Master's degree level or higher, certified midwives and nurse-midwives manage normal pregnancy, birth and newborn care independently. We can order lab tests, sonograms and offer epidural anesthesia in the hospital setting when needed. In 2009 about 12,000 certified nurse-midwives delivered 313,516 babies – 7.6 percent of all births and 11.3 percent of vaginal births. (One-third of U.S. births are now Cesareans.) We also provide primary well-woman care including prescribing contraception, treating sexually transmitted infections, performing Pap smears and breast exams.

Most of us worked as nurses before becoming midwives, but that is no longer a requirement in some states. We are not supervised by doctors, but consult and collaborate with them when abnormalities arise. Midwives take many of the same courses as doctors: biology, anatomy and physiology, genetics, statistics, normal and abnormal labor and birth, psychology and pharmacology. Physicians deal with disease and injury. Their education in the normal is largely to prepare them for the abnormal: when pathogens or tumors invade the body and the immune system is overwhelmed, when organs do not function properly, when bones break, blood is lost or tissues tear.

In training midwives probably spend more time studying normal pregnancy and birth, with their many variations, than medical students. That is the heart of our practice. We do not view the normal mainly as preparation for the interesting complications. The ordinary miracle of life is interesting enough.

Midwifery is a profession based on healthy processes. Pregnancy is not a disease; birth does not routinely require medical or surgical intervention. Pregnancy complications do occur. Surgery may be needed to preserve health, save lives. We are ever on the alert for problems and welcome the expertise and skills of obstetricians in these situations. But our philosophy emphasizes "high touch, low tech": let labor begin on its own and proceed at its own pace as long as mother and baby are doing well. We trust birth rather than try to control it. Science supports this approach: women cared for by midwives have outcomes as safe as those who are treated by obstetricians but with far fewer interventions, such as inductions or Cesareans, have less need for epidural anesthesia, are more likely to breastfeed and feel more satisfied with their childbirth experience.

During my career as a midwife I delivered the babies of some 1,400 mothers and cared for many more thousands of pregnant and laboring women, as well as those seeking contraception.

Every patient taught me something. Some taught me about confronting fear, pain and adversity; many shared the joy, wonder and triumph of giving birth. Some showed me aspects of their culture or religion. And some held up a mirror which revealed my own strengths and failings.

CHAPTER 3

Cherry blossom time

The world is covered in pink. Fallen petals of cherry blossoms cover the grass; tree boughs bend under the weight of blooms. Children scoop up handfuls of petals to throw in the air, laughing under the pink rain. A young mother brushes petals off her daughter's blond braids. The little girl's younger brother does somersaults in the petal-strewn grass. Sometimes, his head and feet on the ground, small bottom in the air, he cannot quite get the momentum to complete the flip; the mother gives him a push and over he goes. Then she brushes petals off his face and clothes as they laugh together.

That young mother is me. It is the first week of May 1967. The little girl is my 4-year-old daughter Sara. The boy, my son Adam, will soon be 3. The esplanade of flowering cherry trees was planted here in the Brooklyn Botanical Garden two years before my birth. I am 23 years old and so carelessly innocent that I do not even realize how happy I am.

In those days I only cared about three things. The small world of my husband and children. The civil rights movement that stirred a passion for justice in my heart. Opposition to the war in Vietnam with its unimaginable violence and horror. Nothing else mattered. I know I cooked meals – shopping at the Associated supermarket on Saturday mornings and dragging a cart full of groceries home while my husband John played with our babies. But I cannot remember a single menu. I know I sewed dresses for my daughter, baked brownies, and read to the children every night at bedtime. But I cannot remember buying clothes for myself or furniture for our apartment. Those were unimportant. My family, civil rights and the war were the trinity of my young life.

* * *

Five years earlier, as a teenage bride and soon-to-be mother, I had listened, enthralled, to the birth stories of my husband's Aunt Clara. She had delivered her son at home in 1933 attended by a midwife, her Aunt Josie.

"A midwife can do so many things to make you feel comfortable," Clara told me. "And Josie was trained at a famous school for midwives." That must have been the Bellevue Hospital School for Midwives. The students, like Josie who came from Sicily, were mainly immigrants. This first professional midwifery school in the country operated in New York City from 1911 to 1936.

Clara's story was fascinating but her attitude was completely foreign to me. Why would anybody want to have her baby at home, right in the bed where she slept? It seemed so messy, old fashioned, practically medieval. Why not go to the hospital, like women normally do?

When my two babies were born in the hospital I learned the down side of such care. I had to fight not to be drugged, put to sleep or tied down, was unable to hold my newborns until hours later, and my husband was barred from the delivery room. Prenatal care consisted of being weighed by a nurse and having the doctor feel my belly and listen to the baby's heartbeat with a stethoscope. Mothers were sternly warned to avoid salt and not to gain more than 15 pounds during the entire nine months, recommendations not based on scientific research and later discarded. There was little opportunity, and no encouragement, to ask questions.

"Let me worry about that," one obstetrician told me when I asked a question about my pregnancy. I don't recall the question, but I certainly remember his answer. He was not being unusually arrogant or unresponsive. In the early 1960s doctors made all the decisions and were not expected to share their reasons or methods with patients, whether men, women or especially children. It was common to withhold a serious diagnosis, particularly cancer, from the patient if, in the physician's opinion, he or she "couldn't handle it." Families rarely dared disobey doctor's orders.

Luckily for me a friend who had recently given birth lent me her copy of *Painless Childbirth Through Psychoprophylaxis*. This book described the method of childbirth preparation developed in the former Soviet Union and later popularized by French obstetrician Fernand Lamaze. English-speaking audiences were introduced to these techniques for reducing childbirth pain in Marjorie Kamel's 1959 book, *Thank You, Dr. Lamaze.*

Being psychologically prepared for labor and able to remain conscious during birth was transformational. I felt a strength and power that no other experience could match.

Years afterward I came across an article about contemporary midwives in a magazine, picked up by chance in a dentist's office. I immediately knew, "That's what I want to do." I would bring empathetic and empowering care to birthing mothers, my hands and voice the gentle instruments I could offer my sisters in their most vulnerable, and most powerful, moments. The drive to become a midwife impelled me on a long, bumpy road to my goal.

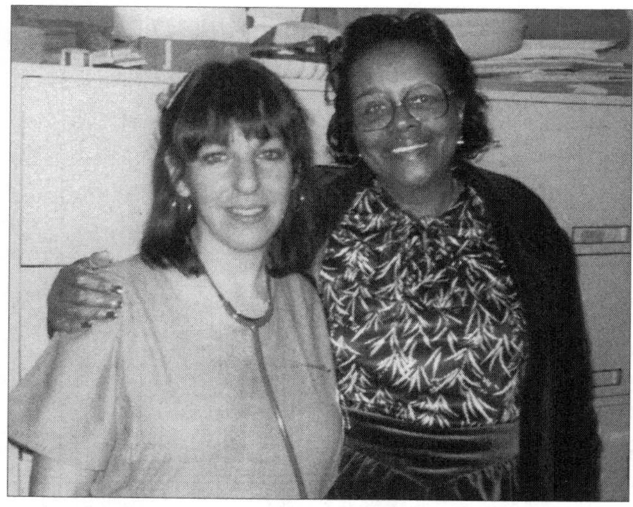

Author, left, Ms. Wiggins, Licensed Practical Nurse, right, Bellevue circa 1982. Ms. Wiggins taught me sterile technique: how to scrub in, set up the operating room for Cesarean surgery and hand instruments to the doctors. Photo: Author

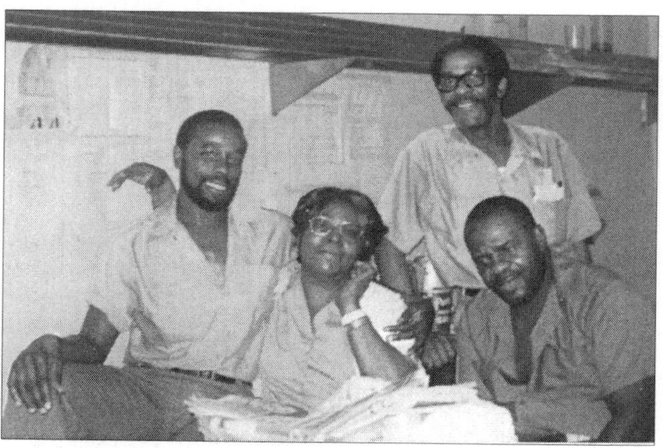

Housekeepers at Bellevue, circa 1981. Photo: Author

Facing page: Bellevue Hospital front gate, 2011.
Photo: Jim.Henderson

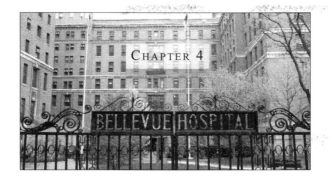

Bellevue

In 1973 I entered the program at the City University of New York's Hunter-Bellevue School of Nursing as the first step toward my dream of becoming a midwife. My husband John did not understand my drive to do this. Our children were then nine and ten years old. My husband had to take over many of the family duties that I abandoned for my studies. We moved from Brooklyn to Stuyvesant Town in Manhattan a few years later to be closer to my school, uprooting then teenaged Sara and causing a first serious mother-daughter fight. At times it seemed as if our marriage could not endure the strain of my new direction. It did not help that couples were breaking up all around us in those years. But the gravitational pull of our merged history and family bonds kept John and me together as I graduated from nursing school and began working on the maternity unit at Bellevue Hospital.

* * *

Bellevue is the oldest hospital in the United States, opened in 1736 and operating continuously until flooding from Hurricane Sandy forced it to evacuate about 500 patients on October 31, 2012 and close temporarily. Although often popularly regarded primarily as a psychiatric center, it has dozens of departments from AIDS and ambulatory surgery to cardiology and pediatrics. Injured firefighters and police officers are rushed to its renowned emergency room and trauma center.

During 2011 Bellevue admitted more than 31,000 patients to its 800 beds; its outpatient clinics handled more than half a million visits. The Emergency Department treated 125,798 people. Midwives attended more than one-third of the 1,785 births. Patients are served regardless of their ability to pay.

There have been many firsts at Bellevue. In 1799 it established the first maternity ward in the U.S. After the Civil War Bellevue doctors helped develop New York City's sanitary code, the first in the world. In 1873 it opened the first nursing school in this country based on Florence Nightingale's methods. When the first pavilion for the insane was opened on hospital grounds in 1879 it was considered revolutionary. The hospital's current state-of-the-art building opened in 1973, the year I entered its nursing program.

Obstetrics nurse, 1979–1982

The Bellevue nurse's cap was a sheer white pillbox, its frilly sides contained by a thin band of black velvet ribbon. It was ridiculous, but did serve one function: informing patients that the wearer was a nurse. My hair was parted down the middle, braided and pinned up in a crown. Hair pins attached the cap to the braids in a slightly shaky confection. To me the look was simultaneously old fashioned and professional. In a white polyester uniform, with matching pantyhose and shoes, I half felt like an imposter pretending to be a nurse. Too bad my recent search through old papers did not yield the Bellevue ID badge with the photo that showed me in this outfit.

Hospitals are scary places full of strange sights, sounds, smells and their own special language.

What do you look at in a patient's room? The monitor broadcasting the heart rhythm in neon green on a gray screen? The fluid slowly dripping into a vein? The plastic bag of amber-colored urine hanging from the bedframe? The flowers and balloons from well-wishers? The gravy-covered mashed potatoes congealing on the dinner tray? The anxious person under the sheets?

What do you listen to? The conversation going on behind the curtain? The beeps of the machines? The sound of someone urinating into a bedpan? The jargon of doctors and nurses? The codes being announced over the public address system, disguised as colors but meaning that a patient has stopped breathing or a heart has stopped beating?

Do the odors of alcohol or feces make you grimace? Are you relieved that the only thing you smell is floor wax or the food on meal trays rattling down the corridor on a big metal cart?

The easiest thing to do is take refuge in the one familiar and non-threatening object in the room – the television set mounted high on the wall like an all-seeing eye. It draws every eye and ear to its ceaseless motion and noise so you can avoid the disturbing sights and sounds that fill the rest of the room.

But gradually, whether you are a patient or visitor, this alien world starts to seem normal. And when you work in a hospital it quickly becomes routine. Within weeks Bellevue was just my workaday destination.

In nursing school the professors taught us to care for individual patients, but we never learned how a hospital unit is organized and run on a daily basis – or how to manage caring for eight or ten patients at once. I was a Registered Nurse with a degree as Bachelor of Science in Nursing, but had never worked in a hospital. There was much to learn during those first awkward months as I was oriented to the four divisions of Bellevue's OB/GYN service: gynecology, postpartum, labor and delivery, and the newborn nursery. I watched and listened but avoided asking too many questions that would expose my enormous ignorance. Luckily no patients were harmed by my inexperience.

In the hospital we addressed each other military-style by last name, prefaced by Doctor, Mr., Miss, Mrs. or the recently coined Ms. In the mid-1960s non-professional New York City hospital workers, who were largely African American, had been organized into unions in a drive that was closely linked to the civil rights movement of those years. The dignity demanded by nurses' aides, laundry, cleaning and kitchen staff included being addressed politely, no first names.

My two-syllable surname, Cohen, was shortened to Cone. Twenty years later when I ran into a former Bellevue colleague we instantly reverted to the names we had called each other back then.

"Cone!" she exclaimed.

"Aponte!" I replied.

My first Bellevue assignment was on the postpartum ward, which housed mothers who had just given birth, as well as women having pregnancy complications. Each morning the entire staff gathered in the nurses' station to get reports on patients from the outgoing night shift. Then we would proceed together from room to room, wheeling a large supply cart of linens, and making beds in pairs.

The businesspeople who manage hospitals today would consider having college-educated Registered Nurses changing sheets with nurses' aides inefficient and a terrible waste of money. But it was an opportunity to observe the way patients moved from bed to chair, if their breakfast trays were empty or full, if their sheets were stained with blood – things a nurse would never learn by checking lab results in a computer or popping a pill into the mouth of a patient sitting passively in bed. The way a mother handled a baby showed her readiness, or lack of it, to care for her new child. While making beds we were alerted to one patient's severe postpartum depression and psychosis when we noticed food mashed up on her tray and smeared all over her face. She could be treated before she hurt herself or her infant.

Another advantage of morning bed-making rounds was that nobody injured her back lifting a mattress alone to tuck in the sheets: that is no small thing in occupations like nursing (or hotel housekeeping) with high injury rates. We worked in pairs, one person on each side of the bed. The nurses' aides, who were usually older than the RNs, set the pace: relaxed, steady, highly efficient. The beds, with perfect hospital corners and blankets artfully fan-folded near the foot, were all made up in time for morning coffee break. Inexperienced and always behind on my patient care assignments or paperwork or both, I rarely had time for coffee breaks.

In the afternoons patients and staff members who could get away from their duties all gazed up at wall-mounted televisions to watch the popular soap opera "General Hospital." The infallible (white male) doctors, sexy (all female) nurses, and glamorous patients who never looked sick were the fantasy version of our reality.

One Saturday during morning rounds a resident pointed to the chattering television sets and remarked disdainfully to his colleagues, "This is Bellevue, where the patients watch cartoon shows." I had to bite my tongue not to remind him that he had learned most of what he knew about hands-on medicine from practicing on those same patients. That included excruciating forceps deliveries performed unnecessarily on our mothers so he could hone his skills for future private patients.

Early in my career many co-workers left work one afternoon to attend the funeral of a young nurse who had died of hepatitis from being stuck with a dirty needle after using it to inject a sick child. She never bothered with the time-consuming process of filing a report about the accident, so her family could not even receive any monetary compensation for her death. This taught me to never omit any paperwork that might protect me. And to be extra cautious with needles, a lesson that served me well in the era of AIDS, then spreading silently all around the world but not identified as a disease until June 1981.

* * *

After a month each in postpartum and gynecology I rotated to the newborn nursery and received my first blue cotton scrub dress. These came in three sizes. The 'large' was too skimpy for big women and rode up over their hips to miniskirt proportions. The ties in back, too short to knot together, hung down like twin tails. Size 'medium' was baggy on petite women like me. We pulled the waist ties tight with enough left over to make a big bow in the back. A size 'small' existed in theory, but I never managed to find one. Patch pockets on the front of the skirt could barely accommodate all the paraphernalia a nurse needs to carry to avoid endless trips back and forth to the supply room. Bending forward, sitting down or standing up all risked a cascade of gauze, pens, keys, or notes on scraps of paper. I remember a co-worker's loud "Oh shit!" coming from the bathroom as she leaned over to flush the toilet and saw the ring of keys to her car and apartment swirl down the bowl.

Stamped in five-inch high letters on the seat of the scrub dress was the name of the institution. Some management expert must have believed this would prevent workers from taking home their hospital-issued scrubs. More than three decades later I still have mine.

Working in the nursery with healthy newborns sounds like fun, but I mostly hated it. Taking vital signs, measuring how much formula was left after each feeding, giving morning baths, wheeling babies to their mothers in plastic bassinets on rolling metal carts, writing standard nursing notes. Nothing terrible in that, but Head Nurse H, while capable and caring towards the infants, made my life miserable. Intimidation and humiliation were her managerial techniques. Although not much older than I was, she wore a large winged nursing cap from another era that made her appear huge and imposing in my eyes. Instead of explaining to this brand new nurse exactly what was expected, she gave vague assignments, then pounced when I did not carry them out to her exacting standards.

Of the twenty or so newborns in the nursery there was often one going through withdrawal from the heroin or methadone which his or her mother had used during pregnancy and the fetus shared in the womb. (Crack cocaine had not yet appeared, and women who could afford the expensive powder form were not likely to deliver at Bellevue.)

These babies might be jittery and cry inconsolably. Sucking fiercely at a bottle, but in an uncoordinated manner, they often failed to put on weight. The nurses and aides would swaddle them tightly in flannel receiving blankets as a comfort measure. I am ashamed to say we called them junkie babies.

Sometimes swaddling was not enough and the pediatricians prescribed phenobarbitol, a drug that acts by slowing activity in the brain, to calm the baby and help her go through withdrawal. Once the hospital pharmacy sent the nursery a bottle of adult strength phenobarbitol, many times stronger than the pediatric dosage used for newborns. Luckily, the nurse who drew up the medicine noticed the mistake; the baby might have died if it was given a massive dose meant for an adult. This type of error was still in the news several years ago when the 12-day-old twins of actor Dennis Quaid and Kimberly Buffington received near-fatal adult doses of a blood thinner.

In the nursery I distinguished myself as the slowest and sloppiest at bathing babies and combing their hair into tiny pompadours. Everyone laughed at me when I mentioned that lint in the baby linens always seemed to wind up on the infants' foreheads. From under her starched white cap Ms. H looked down and informed me coldly, "These patients think a piece of white thread on their babies' brows will cure the hiccups."

The only satisfaction I had was holding up naked just-born infants so their families could see them through the glass windows of the nursery. I would always turn the babies around so the happy fathers and grandparents also got a look at the newborn's little buttocks. That made everybody laugh, including me.

After a miserable month in the nursery I was glad to finally reach my destination: Labor and Delivery, where I could begin to prepare for my future career as a midwife. The head nurse there was Ms. Mogk. Her body was stocky but she had the most delicate hands and fingers, which often held a cigarette. Her reddish hair peeped out from under a blue paper shower cap.

"Mogk is fair," was the high praise the staff gave her. Fair was a head nurse who distributed the better and worse daily patient care assignments equitably, honored requests for days off, and, come December, scheduled everyone to have time off to celebrate their preferred holiday – either Christmas or New Year's.

On my first day of orientation in Labor and Delivery Mogk looked me up and down.

"Put that nurse's cap in your locker before it lands in a bedpan," she advised, a tiny smile in her eyes. The cap went back into its original small box on a top shelf of my closet and only came out once to appear briefly as a costume in an off-off Broadway production. From then on a blue paper shower cap covered my hair.

I wondered what awful things Mogk had heard about me from my nemesis, Head Nurse H in the Newborn Nursery. But Mogk was fair. If I arrived with a reputation as a dud she ignored it and gave me a chance for redemption. She sensed I was eager to learn and she taught me well. Within months I had proven my competence and she decided to keep me permanently in the labor room, no more rotating around to the other units. When Mogk became confident that I could run Labor and Delivery as the nurse in charge, she scheduled me to work on the weekends she was off.

"If you can change a roll of toilet paper you can do this," was her anxiety-busting introduction to a new task or procedure. With a few flicks of those delicate fingers Mogk could shave off a patient's pubic hair in the short interval between labor pains. With practice – and I got to practice many times each shift – I could do it almost as well.

This perineal shave was abandoned when, finally subjected to scientific research toward the end of the 20th century, it was proven to cause infections rather than prevent them. Several other long-practiced obstetric procedures have also been shown to do more harm than good. These include episiotomy, a cut made into the area between the vagina and rectum to widen the vaginal opening just before the baby is born, and until fairly recently a routine procedure at most births.

And we no longer strap women onto the delivery table with thick leather bands around the wrists and ankles. It wasn't a study that ended the use of these soft shackles, but a women's movement that questioned, defied, and eventually eliminated such degrading and harmful medical practices.

My dream was to become a midwife, but I had never actually met one until I began my rotation to Labor and Delivery and had the good fortune to work with three wonderful midwives. Karen Burgin, Tam Le and Kathy Kowalski lavished loving and competent care on patients and showed me what it really meant to practice this profession, even under the less than ideal conditions at a busy public hospital where educating residents and medical students seemed to take priority over patient-centered care.

Spanish was the first language of many patients so I made an effort to pick up a working vocabulary of birth-related words and phrases. Speaking to a woman in her mother tongue seemed one way to reduce her anxiety during the stress of labor and birth. My speech mimicked the way I heard Spanish pronounced, startling some listeners with my Puerto Rican inflections. "Mi hija" (my daughter) and "mi amor" (sweetheart) were endearments I copied in addressing patients.

After completing orientation to all the units on the 9th floor, nurses had to swing between the 8 a.m. and midnight shifts, a month on each rotation. Nights were torture for me. Despite being blessed with the ability to sleep almost any place or any time – including on the eight-inch-wide bench in the locker room during a 3 a.m. lunch break – my body and mind were never quite right during the months of nights.

The midnight shift also was the most understaffed, even though as many babies were born then as during days. To me the night nursing supervisors seemed lazy and unhelpful. Most of them had not touched a patient in years; I suspected they got into management to avoid doing hands-on care.

"Do the best you can," they responded uselessly when we pleaded for more staff or some crucial piece of equipment. And Miss R, head nurse on nights in Labor and Delivery, had a well-deserved reputation for meanness toward both staff and patients. Even the doctors were afraid of her. To escape rotating to nights, I requested a permanent assignment to evenings, starting at 3:30 p.m. and ending at midnight.

Looking back, it was a mistake to work evenings. My children seemed to be navigating their teen years well, but did I really know? I was not around in the afternoons when they got home from school, did their homework, hung out with friends.

At year end each shift celebrated Christmas with a party featuring home-cooked specialties from the workers' different cuisines. Jamaicans brought curried goat; Puerto Ricans contributed roast pork and rice and beans; Filipinas made rice noodle dishes and sweet, dense cakes of cassava and coconut; African Americans cooked chicken and macaroni and cheese. Those of us who didn't cook contributed sodas or store-bought desserts. Except for a single square-bottomed bottle of Manischewitz Kosher Concord Grape wine there was no alcohol, at least none openly displayed. People sipped the sweet deep-purple drink from tiny paper medicine cups. I always wondered who brought it, and how it got to be popular among my black and Latina co-workers.

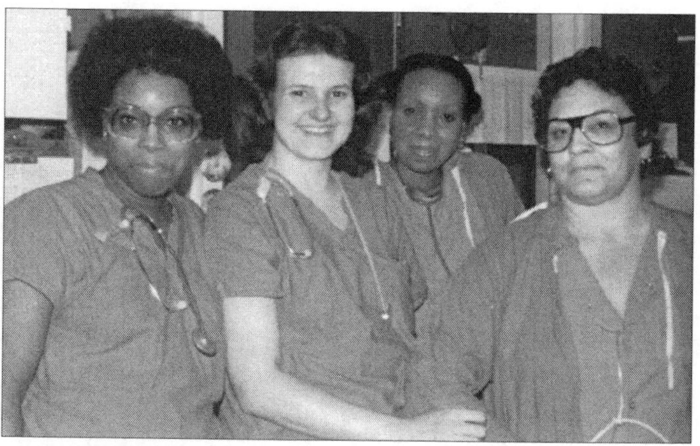

Bellevue Labor and Delivery nurses with midwife Kathy Kowalski, right, circa 1981. Photo: Author

Chapter 5

After

Certain events forever divide life into 'before' and 'after.' When I returned to work following a few days off for Christmas, 1980, my co-workers could see the change in my usually cheerful personality and the pain in my eyes. Nobody pried into my business, nobody asked if I wanted to talk about it. They fed me.

"Cone, you want some fish?" someone might offer. Or, "Like to taste my rice and peas?"

I did not want to talk about it, did not know how to say the words. My 16-year-old son had suffered a mental breakdown and was on a locked psychiatric floor in another hospital. The doctors initially thought his psychosis had been caused by taking LSD and would be temporary. I was never part of the drug culture of the 1960s and didn't even know LSD was still around in 1980. But the hallucinations did not go away. Schizophrenia, a mental illness that often first strikes during adolescence, was the eventual diagnosis.

I wanted my baby back. The doctors needed to do whatever was necessary to drive out the demons that possessed his mind. Psychotherapy, drugs, vitamins, anything – I might even give permission for electroshock if that held out any hope of curing him.

Adam had been born in 1964. The Civil Rights movement was at its peak. I heard the radio news announce that President Lyndon B. Johnson was expanding the Vietnam War while I was nursing my baby boy. "A Hard Day's Night" by the Beatles and Bob Dylan's "The Times They Are a-Changin'" were released that year; The Supremes' "Baby Love" hit the top of the charts. "My Fair Lady" and "Mary Poppins" shared most of the Academy Awards in 1964, beating out Stanley Kubrick's apocalyptic comedy "Dr. Strangelove."

At the time of his breakdown my son was 16 years old, downy-cheeked with long, light brown hair. He was the youngest person on a locked ward of decrepit men and women. Under fluorescent lights gender differences were nearly obliterated by identical hospital gowns, matted hair and zombie-like gait. I offered a non-believer's surreptitious prayers pleading with God to make Adam well again. The medical profession had little to offer. Demonic possession seemed as good an explanation as the scientific theories still in vogue in 1980.

"Schizophrenia is believed to be caused by bad mothering," a young psychiatrist caring for Adam told me. His eyes avoided mine and his face flushed slightly as he delivered this verdict.

I visited Adam every afternoon before my evening labor room shift. In the dayroom people stared vacantly at the television: "Iran Hostage Crisis: Day 430-something" splashed across the screen. A ping-pong table stood mostly unused. Pajama-clad patients wandered in and out asking for a light for cigarettes which they held in trembling, nicotine-stained fingers. Visitors looked nearly as pathetic as the inmates, just dressed in street clothes instead of hospital gowns. I have little memory of our conversations during those visits. Perhaps there was not much talk, as we looked at one another across an abyss of grief for a young life forever changed and diminished. My son, my baby, had been stolen by a terrible disease. My failure as a mother was exposed to the whole world.

There were few anti-psychotic medications available in those years. Haldol caused my son's body to become rigid, saliva foamed in his mouth. His eyes were dark with terror. The doctor on duty shrugged it off as a common side effect, finishing up some paperwork that he considered more important before ordering an antidote. Prolixin caused dry mouth and tremors. Thorazine made patients sluggish, their paper slippers rustling as they shuffled along the corridor.

"I'm not crazy," Adam insisted, "These pills they make me take are the problem."

Going to work was a relief. My labor room duties were demanding and temporarily crowded out the overwhelming fear, helplessness and guilt that dominated my thoughts and feelings when I was not busy. Chit-chat with co-workers dragged me out of isolation. Caring for patients made me feel useful. At midnight I could go home and collapse into sleep. But waking up the next morning did not end the nightmare.

The whole family was devastated. Our older daughter was now away at college, left to suffer on her own as we concentrated all our attention on the sick child. My husband and I could barely look at one another, seeing in the other's face the image of our son and the mirror of our own pain. Only in the dark could we come together for comfort. Adam's grandparents and great-grandparents were stricken, baffled, had no idea what to do. Suggestions from relatives and friends that were meant to be helpful felt like an attack on us for failing to do enough. The stigma surrounding mental illness deepened our isolation and shame.

Walking past Adam's high school I hated the students clustered outside, talking and laughing, normal kids. I wished one of them had gotten sick instead of my son.

Drugs and alcohol were not part of my world but coffee and cigarettes became my friends, giving a brief moment of relief as I sipped, inhaled and forgot. You could smoke any place then. On psychiatric wards the staff handed out cigarettes to patients as rewards, bribes and something to do in the empty hours of empty lives.

Every bit of energy was consumed by Adam's illness: fighting with the doctors to formulate a treatment plan, fighting with Adam to accept it, fighting with the insurance company. My dream of becoming a midwife was put on hold for several years.

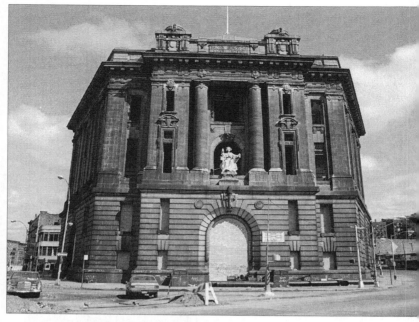

Above, abandoned Bronx County Courthouse, 1980, along the BX 55 bus route.
Photo: Lisa Kahane, NYC
© All Rights Reserved

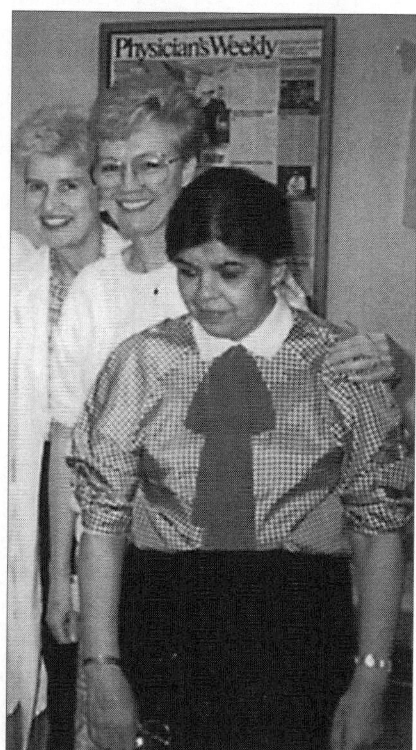

Left to right: Sr. Maureen, Mary Widhalm, Dr. Khakoo, Lincoln Hospital, 1990.
Photo: Author

Laboring:

CHAPTER 6

Lincoln Hospital, 1983–90

As commuter trains rush from Grand Central Terminal and Penn Station toward suburbs north and east of New York City, Lincoln Hospital is the unadorned red brick building that looms over the tracks just after trains cross the Harlem River from Manhattan to the Bronx. This was where I worked from 1983, fresh out of the SUNY Downstate nurse-midwifery program in Brooklyn, until 1990. During those years I cared for thousands of pregnant women and girls, and delivered some 800 babies. From time to time when in need of a smile I picture all those babies holding hands in a long line, from the youngest to the oldest. Would that line be long enough to encircle the new Yankee Stadium a mile away from the hospital? My mathematician husband calculates it would. Now my babies are all grown up, many with babies of their own. Some, I fear, have already died.

* * *

The moon was high in the autumn sky as I walked from the 149th Street subway station to Lincoln Hospital. This was my first night shift as a midwife in Labor and Delivery. I was terrified of the life and death responsibility of caring for pregnant women and delivering babies. A long road of ten years had brought me here. This was the profession that felt so right for me, that I worked so hard to enter, sometimes neglecting my family along the way. Unsure of my newly acquired skills, my mind flashed back to Bellevue. As a nurse it was easy to second-guess and criticize the doctors whose orders I followed. As a midwife, I felt the full weight of making and carrying out patient care decisions. It was humbling and made me less quick to condemn others when they performed like fallible human beings.

Back in the newborn nursery I was the novice nurse who couldn't get the babies assigned to her washed and combed fast enough. Now I was a novice midwife and my responsibilities went far beyond baths and baby hairdos; lives and health were at stake.

Only knowing that I was mentored by experienced midwives Mary Widhalm and Angelina Chambers gave me the courage to enter the building, put on scrubs, fling a stethoscope around my neck, and push open the swinging doors to the labor room. With Mary holding one hand and Angie the other, I took baby steps forward. They didn't let go of my hands until they knew I was ready to safely care for patients. The sheer volume of births at Lincoln gave me plenty of experience in a short time. Slowly, tentatively, our hands unclasped. Then I was walking on my own.

But sometimes I stumbled. During the first months at Lincoln one of my prenatal patients suffered a stillbirth. Death seems especially hard in maternity care: it is so unexpected, the opposite of the anticipated new life. A pregnant woman dreams of her child. Her baby has lived for many months in a mother's body and imagination by the time it is born. A stillbirth is not only the death of a baby but of all those dreams, that imagined life. It does not comfort a mother to tell her "It's easier to lose the baby now, before you knew her and loved her." The knowing and the loving happen long before the birth.

I was devastated. Could I have done something to prevent this tragedy? Staring into the darkness on sleepless nights I was ready, almost, to abandon this profession. Mary, the chief midwife, sat down with me. We reviewed the patient's medical record together.

"Your charting is impeccable," she said. Many others helped me become a midwife but Mary was responsible for my staying a midwife. She would not let me quit.

Months passed. The moon in the summer sky over the Bronx was the same as last fall, but I was different. Adrenalin still pumped through my body as I entered Labor and Delivery. But it was no longer all driven by fear: I felt challenged but ready. I had mastered procedures and techniques, gained confidence in my skills. The paperwork no longer baffled me. I had figured out which doctors to trust and which ones to avoid, which nurses cared about the patients and which ones just wanted get through their shift with minimal effort. I'd learned how to maneuver a bit around a system that isolated a laboring woman at the time she most needed human contact.

Within a few years I had accumulated enough experience to become a clinical instructor, doing hands-on teaching of medical and midwifery students. I gave a class on normal birth to medical students. A calico cloth doll, complete with umbilical cord and placenta, a plaster pelvis and a series of plastic circles simulating cervical dilatation were my props.

Long before ethics courses became standard in medical schools we discussed the students' responsibility toward patients and the morality of learning on living human beings what can first be practiced on an inanimate model. The doctors-to-be appreciated the chance to learn hand maneuvers for delivering a baby with my doll. Clinical midwifery education is based on safely practicing with an experienced teacher at one's side to guide the learner, and if necessary take over if the student is not up to the task. Ongoing feedback between teacher and learner is part of the process. It is far different from the "see one, do one, teach one" approach of traditional physician training.

Technical skills that must be mastered by diligent practice are essential. My goal was also to teach students to view a situation from the patient's perspective. "Always listen to the patient," was my mantra, learned from wise midwife professor, Lily Hsia.

A third-year med student I will call Robert was upset. He had done all the "scut work" – admission forms, starting an IV, drawing blood – and was eager to do his first delivery. The patient assigned to his care was in labor with her third child. We expected a relatively quick and easy birth. But he missed his chance: the baby was born without his help.

"What happened?" I asked Robert.

"She was 5 centimeters dilated when I examined her," he said. "A minute or two later she started saying 'the baby is coming.' But it seemed way too soon. I was explaining this to her when she gave a big grunt. Then I heard the baby crying from under the sheets."

Always listen to the patient. No laboring woman ever misled me with her urgent "the baby is coming!"

Never enough

In 2011 Lincoln Hospital logged 429,060 outpatient visits, saw 155,298 patients in the emergency room, and delivered 2,461 babies according to data from New York City's Health and Hospitals Corporation. When I worked there, we delivered twice as many. Often all six labor rooms were occupied; any additional patients labored on stretchers in the hallway. During a typical 12-hour shift I would attend two or three births, care for twice that many women in labor, and triage others to determine whether they could be sent home or needed admission. There never seemed to be enough doctors, nurses, midwives, space or equipment. On a busy day – or night – the waiting area was full of patients, pacing and groaning as they waited their turn to be seen. I would look around to see if any of the patients seemed close to giving birth, and bring her to the triage room ahead of turn.

"Sorry, mothers," I would say to the others, "I know some of you were here before her, but we need to take care of the most urgent patients first." The women understood. Sometimes they would tell me, "Check her," pointing to another patient who appeared more in need of attention. I could understand when they spoke about me in Spanish, saying "At least she explains to us what's happening."

During my years there the hospital served a million people in the surrounding South Bronx and upper Manhattan. The population of this area was largely Puerto Rican and African American with a growing number of Mexican immigrants and others from Central and South America. Spanish was spoken more than English.

The maternity service was on the fifth floor. It included the labor and delivery unit, postpartum ward, and newborn nursery. Lincoln also had medical, surgical, pediatric and psychiatric departments, each with its own inpatient floor as well as outpatient clinics. Separate emergency rooms treated adults, children and psychiatric patients. People suffering asthma attacks – a common malady in the Bronx – went directly to a special asthma room for treatment to ease their wheezing. Lincoln also pioneered in using acupuncture for drug detoxification.

I once came across an unofficial newsletter written and xeroxed by some doctors. One article discussed the dilemma of the psychiatrist who had to determine which of the emergency room patients claiming to be suicidal really was in danger of killing him- or herself versus who was there seeking shelter and something to eat. The writer suggested serving a tray of food to all the patients. Those who are truly suicidal, he wrote, will be too depressed to bother feeding themselves, and need to be admitted. Those who are merely destitute will eat every morsel, and can safely be discharged. He said this method may appear to come from *Alice in Wonderland*, but under the conditions existing at this overwhelmed hospital the food tray test was a crude but fairly reliable way to decide which patients truly needed the limited resources available. I no longer have this newsletter, but the gist of the article was unforgettable.

Teen Clinic

Lincoln's prenatal program for teenagers had been started by our chief midwife, Mary Widhalm, in the early 1970s when teen pregnancy rates were very high. Our girls were young and healthy;

most did not smoke, drink or use drugs. But some complications are more prevalent in adolescents, especially pre-eclampsia, which involves high blood pressure, swelling of the face and hands, and protein in the urine. It can progress to seizures, called eclampsia, possibly causing stillbirth and even maternal death.

In addition to the potential health risks of motherhood at such a young age was the greater social risk of dropping out of school, losing the chance at education and skills needed for employment.

Teen Clinic started at 4 o'clock. The message was "go to school first, then come for your check-up." As the girls arrived we weighed them, checked their blood pressure and urine and sent them to the lab if blood work was needed. Family members and the babies' fathers were always welcome. Then everyone squeezed into a conference room for a class. We had no slick educational materials and an informal curriculum encompassing pregnancy, birth, baby care, breastfeeding, sex education and contraception. Our birth video was so old the characters wore bell-bottoms and hairstyles from the 1960s.

All the midwives took turns teaching. We encouraged the audience to ask – and answer – questions.

"Can a girl get pregnant the first time she has sex?" Several who once thought the answer was 'no' sat there with big bellies.

"Does having sex during pregnancy help you have an easier birth?"

"Do birth control pills give women cancer?"

"Will nursing the baby make my titties fall down?"

After class came the check-ups. Each girl had her own midwife who cared for her throughout pregnancy. Patients rarely missed their visits, and if they did we would call them to find out why. This continuity of care, personal attention and group health education was unique to Teen Clinic.

"The midwives spoil those girls," was the verdict of people who were used to working in a conveyor-belt system geared to speedy patient visits with any available doctor rather than a long-term relationship with a "private" midwife. But Dr. Reguero, the head of obstetrics, credited Mary and the midwives with lowering infant mortality in the South Bronx. And the chief of pediatrics, Dr. Rajagowda, frequently told us, "The high-risk mommies need midwives too."

BX 55 bus

The BX 55 bus carried me from Lincoln through the gutted midsection of the South Bronx to the Maternity, Infant Care, and Family Planning Projects (MIC) clinic at 1826 Arthur Avenue where I saw prenatal and contraceptive-seeking patients.

Its route passed burnt out buildings, empty lots strewn with debris and an abandoned octagonal court house, blackened with soot, where a statue of Justice holding her scales sat whitely on a high pedestal overlooking the gray landscape.

Storefront churches named Solid Rock Baptist Church, Greater Evangelical Mission, First Church of Deliverance, Tabernacle of Prayer dotted the route. Billboards in vacant lots mostly advertised cigarettes and expensive brands of liquor. One sign promised, "Jesus makes house calls."

In some of the abandoned tenements empty windows had been covered over with sheet metal painted to look like real windows, complete with curtains and flower pots, part of an effort to make the Bronx look less grim during the years Ed Koch was mayor.

"Isn't it dangerous?" people often asked when they heard where I worked. They might even back away physically, as if being close to me might imperil them. They only knew this part of the city through negative stereotypes in the media. But I felt safe in a neighborhood where women waved and called out "hola doctora" as I traveled on foot and by public transportation between the hospital and clinic.

At East Tremont Avenue I got off the bus and walked uphill past Crotona Park toward the tan building that housed MIC. I had been working there for several years before I noticed that from the top of the hill the Empire State Building was visible in clear weather. From here it seemed like part of a different world.

Mary Widhalm, chief midwife

Mary was born at home on a farm in Nebraska shortly before World War II. She was near the middle of eleven sisters and brothers. When we worked together it never occurred to me to ask her how or why she became a midwife. In my mind Mary had always been a midwife, wise and experienced, from her first breath. It was not until recently, both of us now retired, that I found out about her journey to our profession.

We met in a small cafe close to her apartment on Manhattan's Upper West Side soon after the New Year of 2013. With blue eyes and short blond-gray hair Mary looked no older than when we had last worked together twenty plus years ago. A soft peach-colored shirt complemented her fair complexion; dangling purple earrings gave pizzazz to her outfit. Over mediocre coffee she shared the story of her younger self while boisterous students from a nearby school swirled around our table.

"I always wanted to be a religious [nun] and I liked to sew. After high school I took my vows and was assigned to sewing everyday garments like habits or aprons. From there I might advance to sewing and embroidering more elaborate liturgical robes. After a year or two the mother superior told me, 'Mary, you should use your head more. We are sending you to college to study nursing.'

"'Oh shit,' I thought. I did not want to be a nurse, but had taken vows of obedience, so off I went. I hated it. Orthopedics, with weights for traction and heavy casts – I might as well be back on the farm, pitching bales of hay in the fields. Psychiatry was horrible – electroshock and insulin shock were the treatments then. I looked forward to pediatrics, working with children. But when I got there, I had to teach a mother to give her six-year-old insulin shots. The child was crying, the mother hated me for making her do it. Awful.

"Finally, I got to maternity care. That saved me. Nurses managed women in labor; the doctor was just called for the delivery.

Heaven help you if you called him too soon and he had to hang around waiting for the mother to give birth.

"I first read about midwives in a little booklet published by Ethicon, the company that manufactured suture material. That sent me on a search to find out about midwifery education programs. I wrote to all of them and got a letter back from New York Medical College. At that time it was located in the old Flower Fifth Avenue Hospital on 106th Street and Fifth Avenue in Manhattan. They offered me a full scholarship, plus a stipend for living expenses and money for books! I got permission to go – on the condition that I live in a convent. I found a convent right on West 97th Street. A bus that traveled through Central Park took me from the convent to right near the hospital. They warned me never to go into the park.

"I loved school. Microbiology was wonderful, chemistry even better. We studied all the sciences in the same classes as medical students."

After becoming a midwife Mary asked to be released from her vows in order to practice her new profession fully, including counseling about and providing contraception to women who needed it. She began working at Lincoln in the early 1970s. I was lucky to have her as chief midwife, mentor and friend when she hired me in 1983.

In our interactions I only saw Mary's soft side, but she was hard as nails when it came to standing up for her patients, her midwives or her principles.

"Absolutely not!" She would put her foot down, perhaps when somebody in the Obstetrics Department wanted the midwives to do more "scut" work and fewer births, or a bureaucratic nurse administrator mistakenly insisted that all our orders had to be co-signed by a physician.

She was no longer a nun when we worked together but a patient described Mary's gentle care this way: "Being examined by Ms. Widhalm is like having your Pap test done in heaven." She would chat about a woman's ring or bracelet or the color of her nail polish, completely distracting the patient from the vaginal exam she skillfully performed at the same time.

My mentor taught me a trick for delivering a baby whose cord is wrapped around its neck. This is fairly common and usually is not dangerous, although people always worry that the cord will choke the baby. Remember that the unborn infant does not breathe air through the windpipe into its lungs. He or she gets oxygen from blood flowing through the umbilical cord. The potential danger is that, with one or more loops wrapped tightly around the neck, oxygen flow through the cord will be impeded. If this happens it is the baby that "chokes" the cord, rather than the cord choking the baby.

When delivering a baby we always check for a cord around the neck once the head is out. If we feel a cord, and cannot simply loop it over the head, the textbook procedure is to clamp it in two places and cut between the clamps before delivering the shoulders and body. Sometimes the baby is coming so quickly there is no time for this clamp and cut procedure. The "somersault maneuver" was Mary's solution.

"Just keep the baby's head close to the mother's perineum and let its body somersault out," she explained. "You can unwrap the cord after the baby is completely delivered." I practiced on our calico doll to perfect the hand motions and successfully performed the somersault maneuver at several births.

Labor room morning rounds

"The board" in Labor and Delivery was a large chalkboard that listed all the patients. A typical entry included the patient's room number, age, due date, previous births, cervical dilatation, time her bag of waters ruptured, estimated weight of the baby, medications being administered and actual or potential complications.

Every shift started at board turnover with the outgoing staff giving reports about the patients to those coming on duty. It was important to know the status of all the patients, not just those assigned to one's care. In case of an emergency everybody needed to know where they would be most useful – lending a hand in the crisis situation or making sure the other patients were not neglected during the emergency.

The board was located just inside the swinging double entry doors to the labor unit. Across from it was the ward clerk's desk where patients signed in. At some point, I don't remember in which year, this registration area was encased in bullet-proof glass, like the cash register in a Bronx liquor store. Women had to shout their name, medical record number and the reason they were there through a slot to the clerk at the desk. The slot was level with the seated clerk's face, putting it at about belly-height for the person standing in front. A mother in labor had to bend way down and twist her head so her mouth faced the slot.

After board turnover I would go to meet all the laboring patients and evaluate them myself. I did not want to rely on possibly incomplete notes from the previous night. There were six single-bed labor rooms. If those were full, additional patients lay on stretchers in the long corridor that led to the three delivery rooms. When administration decided that stretchers in the hallway violated some regulation we changed to doubling patients up in the labor rooms. Two patients in a room left barely enough space for the staff to maneuver between the beds, fetal monitors and poles holding intravenous fluids.

In the morning I would help laboring mothers climb out of bed and walk to the bathroom. Being able to urinate in the toilet, rather than on a bedpan, wash up and brush their teeth helped patients' morale. Lying on her back is the worst and most uncomfortable position for labor, and a full bladder can impede progress. Sometimes these simple actions – getting out of bed, walking around, urinating – helped the baby descend in the pelvis. Often mothers gave birth soon afterwards. I didn't care if some of the nurses and doctors thought my methods were a bit weird.

Many of the women had been alone for hours, except for an occasional blood pressure check by a nurse or vaginal exam by a doctor. Research shows that a caring person accompanying a woman makes labor shorter and safer. But relatives were only allowed to stay with patients if they had attended childbirth classes and had a certificate to prove it. The midwives taught these classes and made sure all our teen patients had certificates. We kept a supply of blank certificates that we would fill out on the spot if needed to enable a spouse, mother or friend to stay at the bedside. Nobody needs a month of classes to hold a laboring woman's hand. But even with certificates family members were barred from two-patient rooms.

The hardest part of my rounds was leaving a patient.

"No me dejes solita" or "Don't leave me all alone" each woman would plead. Even more than relief from pain, they craved the comforting presence of another human being. I promised to come back after checking the other patients. On busy days it took a long time before I could return. Sometimes my promise was just a hopeful lie.

"Do you have children?" laboring women often wanted to know. Their question was a polite way of asking if I had shared their experience and knew firsthand what they were going through. They sought a bond, a visceral connection to another woman who had also given birth.

On rounds one morning I noticed the small size of a woman's abdomen as she lay on a stretcher in the hallway. Alarmed that she might be in labor with a dangerously premature baby, I lifted the sheet to check the size of her belly. A full-term newborn lay silent and still between her legs. No time to put on gloves. I unwound two loops of umbilical cord from around his neck and smacked his little feet to get him breathing. It worked. He must have delivered only minutes before I got there.

Had the mother cried out as her baby was born? Was nobody there to respond to her as the night shift disappeared and the day shift had not yet arrived? She was a humble Mexican woman from the countryside. Her first child had been born at home. She knew nothing about how things were done in a hospital. Left alone to labor perhaps she thought that delivering unassisted was another strange, but normal, process in this alien place.

Another morning at about a quarter to eight, coffee in my hands, I peeked into Labor and Delivery before changing into scrubs. On a stretcher in the hallway a woman lay moaning and clutching her belly. Wheeling her into a triage room while asking about her medical history I learned that she was seven months pregnant. No prenatal care. Labor had started a few hours ago but she had not broken her bag of water. Examining her abdomen I felt the tiny fetus, less than three pounds by my estimate. It was in transverse lie (crosswise) in her uterus. From this position the baby cannot be born normally. A Cesarean section is necessary.

A gentle vaginal exam revealed she was fully dilated. Surgery was needed immediately. When the bag of water ruptured – it could happen any second – the umbilical cord might prolapse, or fall out of the cervix. If the cord becomes compressed between the baby's body and the mother's, oxygen to the baby is cut off. He will suffer brain damage or die within minutes.

I popped my head out of the triage room to alert the nurses to set up the operating room for a stat (immediate) Cesarean and to report my findings to the physician on duty. No clerk sat at the desk, no nurses were visible.

"Twenty-eight weeks, transverse lie, fully dilated," I yelled, "we need a stat section." No doctor responded to my shouts. Nobody was there except the patient and me. What should I do? I had to let somebody know about this perilous situation, but I could not leave the patient alone.

The labor unit's door swung open. Arriving at work early, coffee in hand, Mary Widhalm peeked in.

"Mary," I called, "Come here." I gave her a summary of the situation in less than 15 seconds. She stayed with the patient while I ran to the Obstetrics Department office down the hall. I interrupted the doctors' meeting to describe the emergency. Two of them hurried back with me to Labor and Delivery.

Mary had explained to the patient what was going on while starting an intravenous line. Someone called the anesthesiologist and pediatrician. By now the day shift nurses were on duty. One of them wheeled the patient to the operating room, where another nurse scrubbed in to set up the instruments. As soon as the surgeons were ready general anesthesia put the patient to sleep in seconds. An extremely premature baby boy was delivered by Cesarean minutes later. He cried and kicked, but weighed only 2 pounds 7 ounces. The pediatricians took him to Neonatal Intensive Care. I never found out how he did afterward.

The emergency resolved, Mary and I drank our coffee. Mine was tepid, but hers was still warm. It was just a few minutes past 8 a.m. but I felt as if I'd already done a full day's work.

The prisoner

The presence of a policeman outside the Labor and Delivery triage room signaled that the patient awaiting my care was a prisoner. Perhaps she had been brought to Lincoln from the huge high-rise jail called the Bronx House of Detention not far from the hospital, or the complex of court buildings near Yankee Stadium or a local precinct.

The woman was moaning softly to herself as I entered the room. She seemed to be in active labor. But before I could introduce myself, ask about her health history and do a physical exam, the sight of handcuffs shackling her to the gurney made me stop short.

Although trembling inside I summoned my most authoritative "doctor" voice.

"Uncuff her," I told the policeman. "I can't take care of her like this – it's not safe." To soften the request I added, "She won't go anywhere, believe me." Out came the officer's keys and the cuffs disappeared without the fight I was anticipating. But instead of feeling relieved at successfully advocating for humane treatment for my patient, I felt mortified. Witnessing the humiliation the woman suffered made it hard for me to even look at her, even though I was not the one inflicting such cruelty. Her shame became mine.

The prisoner gave birth to a healthy baby and got to hold her newborn for a few minutes before she was shackled again. I don't know what happened to either mother or baby after that. But I thought of my prisoner patient in August, 2009, when Governor David Paterson signed legislation outlawing the shackling of women prisoners during childbirth in New York State. It took a decades-long campaign by the Legal Aid Society and other advocates for pregnant women to end this brutal practice.

Don't push

"Don't push, don't push!" I could hear a deep voice urging the grunting patient before I saw the stretcher come through the doors to the labor area.

"Para one, vertex, bulging perineum," Dr. Modesto told me. In obstetric lingo this means a woman having her second baby and ready to give birth any minute, if not sooner. "Ms. Long is setting up Delivery Room 2 for you." We rushed the stretcher down the corridor to that room. Dr. Modesto returned to his task of triaging and admitting patients. This lady was for me to deliver.

"Blow, blow, blow the pain away," I said to the mother. No time to even ask her name. "Pant like a doggie. Don't push yet. Give me a minute to set up properly to deliver your baby." Useless words. The urge to push is overwhelming at this stage of childbirth. I flung the sheet off the patient to see if the baby's head was starting to emerge. The patient was wearing a body suit that went from her neck and arms, over her big belly, down to between her legs. There were no snaps in the crotch that we could open to let the baby come out. An irrelevant detail that sticks in my memory is the turquoise and green leaf pattern on the fabric.

"Size 6 ½ ok for you?" asked Ms. Long, offering me an open package of sterile gloves.

"Thanks." I grabbed the gloves and pulled them on without taking my eyes off the patient. Spandex could not hold this baby back. It was awkward, but I managed to pull aside the strip of fabric between the mother's legs and help guide the head out with the other hand. The rest of the body needed no help, sliding onto the stretcher in a small puddle of amniotic fluid.

"Boy!" I said over the baby's loud wails.

"Thank you Jesus," the mother cried, lifting her arms, "for giving me back my son… Let me see him."

"Soon as I get him dry and cleaned up," said the nurse.

"My first baby was shot and killed just after he turned one year old," the patient said. "I prayed and prayed to Jesus to give me another son. Now I have my little boy back."

Tears stung my eyes as I helped her peel the body suit down her arms, breasts and across the now deflated abdomen. She lifted her hips off the stretcher so I could slide the garment off beneath her buttocks and over her legs.

"Peroxide should take the blood stains out of this," I said in a husky voice, rolling the wet body suit into a ball and placing it in a corner of the stretcher. I put on another pair of clean gloves to deliver the placenta.

I was not crying for the tragic death of her first little boy, nor over the joyful birth of this baby. Mine were hot tears of jealous rage. She got her baby back, but my son, diagnosed with schizophrenia as a 16-year-old, was lost. Refusing medication, in and out of several psychiatric wards for years, he wandered the streets in the grip of terrifying hallucinations. When was God going to give me back **my** baby?

After completing the patient's chart I described this body suit birth to Dr. Modesto. We laughed together. He was a big man with a deep voice. I liked him. When we worked in prenatal clinic I could hear him from his examining room down the corridor.

"How ya' doing? Everything ok?" Dr. Modesto greeted every patient sociably, in English or Spanish, as he ushered her into his office. The words slid out of one side of his mouth, while the other side worked on a cigar. No glowing tip, no harsh smell of tobacco; the cigar was never lit.

It must have been the GI bill and one of the traditionally black medical schools that allowed Dr. Modesto, a Puerto Rican military veteran, to become a doctor in the era of segregation.

"I love kids," was his explanation for why he chose to become an obstetrician.

He had more than two decades of experience at the time I was struggling through my first year as a midwife. Dr. Modesto described seeing women brought into the emergency room, "Their backs were arched like a bow, rigid, so that only the top of the head and buttocks touched the stretcher they were lying on... That was tetanus," he said, "from an abortion with dirty instruments." He shook his head, as if to clear the image from his mind.

"We don't see that any more, thank God."

Postpartum rounds

I visited all the mothers delivered by a midwife on the previous shift. After introducing myself I would ask how the birth had been. The inevitable answer, whether in English or Spanish, was "normal."

"Yes, you had a normal birth. But how was it for *you*? Was it easy, difficult, long, quick?" I wanted to understand their perception of the experience. Most of the replies were brief, not the vivid story they might tell a mother, sister or friend.

"The only part that hurt was the pains," one of our teens assured me.

"Regular," was a frequent response. In Spanish it had a range of possible meanings: ordinary, normal, so-so, or not so good. Did our patients not want to discuss how they felt? Was it because I was an authority figure to them, however uncomfortable that idea made me feel? Were they intimidated by my interrogation, afraid to give a wrong answer? Or too humble to feel entitled to have an opinion?

"How was the midwife who attended you?" was my next question. Now came the smile and the certain answer, "She stood by me and gave me courage." They almost always used these same words, no matter in which language they were spoken. This was a reaffirmation of the midwives' mission to give our patients confidence in themselves and make every woman feel valued as we guide them safely through birth.

A physical assessment, checking for bleeding, helping get baby to breast and a discussion about contraception and newborn care were part of the postpartum exam. We asked who they lived with, who would help them, who would buy baby clothes and diapers. Did they have a crib, a stroller? Was there heat in the apartment, a refrigerator, food? Sometimes the answers were not reassuring; we would have a social worker interview the patient and try to obtain needed resources. In the 1980s when decent housing was scarce and drugs plentiful in the Bronx, Lincoln had a nursery for "boarder babies" who could not be discharged to unsafe conditions. Volunteers from the community, mostly older women, would feed, diaper and cuddle these infants until the babies went to their parents, or to foster care.

When our postpartum check-ups coincided with visiting hours we got to meet family members: a mother or grandmother spoon-feeding homemade soup to the new mother, a father holding his newborn child with awe and increasing confidence, a sister or friend brushing the patient's hair with slow, loving strokes.

I enjoyed working with almost all my patients. Over the course of six or seven months and a dozen or so prenatal visits, or in the intensity of labor and birth, we bonded. But once in a while there was a patient I did not like. My feeling wasn't based on something she did or said; it was just a matter of chemistry. I was visiting one such patient on my postpartum rounds when I suddenly realized that she did not like me either. It was mutual. What a relief; there was no need to feel guilty. This interaction taught me that I did not have to be a saint who loves everybody, nor Ms. Popularity, loved by all.

Staff lounge

In a large windowed room in Labor and Delivery the staff did paperwork, ate meals, smoked cigarettes or simply sat and relaxed in those rare moments when the flow of patients slowed a bit. A big oval conference table that could seat a dozen people took up most of the room. This was where doctors, nurses, aides and ward clerks shared photos of children, weddings and baby showers. There was often a catalogue of Avon products on the table: when you wash your hands every 15 minutes or so during a 12-hour shift you need a good hand cream. Here I listened to a resident from Turkey singing to himself in a minor key in the pre-dawn hours; learned that a tired nurse had been working as much overtime as she could to earn money to relocate her family to Atlanta, hoping that there her sons would avoid the dangers of the Bronx streets. We were immigrants from around the world and people who had grown up down the block. Some of us lived in the neighborhood and others took the subway or drove cars to places worlds away, although no further geographically than the few miles to Manhattan or the suburbs in Westchester or New Jersey.

The door

Every few years hospitals must go through an accreditation process which includes an on-site inspection. The weeks leading up to this visit were a flurry of activity. Paperwork and protocols were put in order, equipment repaired, supplies that were unobtainable for months suddenly appeared, employees coached in what to say or not say, floors polished, dust excised from hidden corners, illegal coffee pots secreted away. As the date approached we heard rumors that Lincoln's parent organization, New York City's Health and Hospitals Corporation, was sending its "Clean Team" to help us get ready. Lincoln always had a reputation for cleanliness, no matter what other problems the hospital faced, so I wondered about the function of this "Clean Team." On site visit day I found out.

The inspectors were coming. They'd be here in Labor and Delivery within the hour. No food on the unit! Put those paper coffee cups in the trash! Fire doors closed! No patients on stretchers in the hallway!

Two men in maintenance worker uniforms appeared carrying a large piece of wood. They stopped at the entrance to the staff lounge and put down their load. One of them took out an electric drill and plugged the long orange extension cord into an outlet. Then we saw that the board was not just a piece of wood but a door with hinges attached near the top and bottom. The workers screwed the hinges into the wall so the door covered the entrance to the room, as per the rules and regulations of the Joint Commission on Accreditation of Healthcare Organizations.

Soon afterward the inspectors arrived. They did not want to be around women in labor for more than a minute – and quickly left. But the story did not end quite yet. The two workmen returned just minutes later. One of them plugged the drill into the same outlet again. He proceeded to unscrew the hinges, top and bottom, while his partner held the door steady. Then they carried it away, a prop in a play, to reappear in another act.

"That must be the 'Clean Team,'" I realized.

Housekeepers

Birth is messy. There is blood, there is sweat. There is the amniotic fluid surrounding the baby that pours out when the membranes containing it rupture. Hospital gowns and bed sheets get soiled and wet. The staff uses and discards latex gloves. Laundry bags and garbage pails fill up and must be emptied. Floors need to be swept, mopped, then swept and mopped again.

At Lincoln Hospital Mr. Lewis and Mr. Hernandez were housekeepers on the Labor and Delivery service who kept the unit clean. They moved beds, hauled heavy loads of linens and garbage, pushed huge buckets of chlorine-scented mop water. And they did much more than clean. They cared about the patients. They lived in the neighborhood; their wives, daughters and sisters had babies here. If a woman was laboring on a stretcher in the hallway (which happened all the time) and the doctors or medical students were gathered around to examine her, Mr. Lewis or Mr. Hernandez would silently appear with a rolling screen to provide the patient with privacy. And dignity.

Mr. Lewis was of average height, with a broad chest and muscular arms. The music of Jamaica played in his words; a glint of gold winked in his smile. He was a grandfather and wore aviator glasses, but no wrinkles or gray hair gave away his age. In the open V-neck of his green scrub shirt a gold chain with a medal shone against his dark skin. We never stood close enough for me to find out what the medal was.

Mr. Hernandez was Puerto Rican, a young father of three – all born at Lincoln. He had a soft-looking round belly that belied the strength in his hardworking arms.

As they cleaned, Mr. Lewis and Mr. Hernandez listened and observed. They knew the moans of a woman in distress, and the deep grunting sounds of a woman about to deliver. They were extra eyes and ears as we midwives careened from patient to patient, trying to give loving care to too many needy women at once.

"Come quick, sister, check the woman in Room 4," Mr. Lewis or Mr. Hernandez would leave his mop to alert us. Co-workers often called us "sister," a generic title for midwives and nurses used in Britain and the Caribbean. We valued the housekeepers' judgment and would rush to that patient, confirming with our examining fingers what their experienced ears suspected.

"Delivery!" we would call out, pushing the patient's bed or stretcher to the delivery room, hoping that there would be enough nurses on duty to assist at the birth.

One Fourth of July I was working the 8 a.m. to 8 p.m. shift in the labor room. Holidays or weekends meant fewer people at work. When the day nurses went home at 4 p.m. and the afternoon staff came on duty there was not a single regular labor room nurse among them. Management pulled some nurses from other parts of the hospital, sent a few from temporary agencies. There were enough warm bodies to claim that the unit was fully staffed. But these nurses knew nothing about labor and delivery. Having been in a similar position as a nurse I knew they were resentful at being assigned to an unfamiliar area, frightened of making a mistake that might get them in trouble or harm a patient. I glimpsed them nervously huddled in the nurses' station, awaiting instructions from their supervisor. The nurses averted their eyes as Mr. Lewis helped me push Ms. Acevedo's stretcher past them into Delivery Room 1. None of them responded to my urgent call: "We need a nurse to set up this room for a birth. And call pediatrics STAT!"

We needed a pediatrician at the delivery because the patient's amniotic fluid was stained with meconium, a baby's tarry first stool. This puts the baby at risk for aspirating meconium into his lungs with his first breaths, possibly causing pneumonia. The midwife has to suction out the baby's mouth and nose when the head delivers but before the rest of its body is born and she or he starts to cry. After the baby is fully delivered and the umbilical cord is cut the pediatrician takes over to check that there is no meconium below the newborn's vocal cords. [See Notes to the Reader]

Again shouting for assistance, I helped the mother move from the stretcher onto the delivery table. Still no nurse. Then, out of the corner of my eye I saw Mr. Lewis – he was opening the sterile linens, gloves and instruments used for delivery, adding the special suction device needed for clearing meconium from the throat of the newborn and turning on the warmer for the baby bassinet. Having cleaned this delivery room thousands of times he knew exactly what equipment was needed and where to find it. He knew how to open packages and place their contents using sterile technique in order to protect mother and baby from infection. He also knew how many rules he was breaking by acting outside of his job description and by simply being in a room with a naked female patient. As I set up the instruments he laid out I felt him behind me, tying the ties on the back of my sterile gown. When the pediatrician arrived Mr. Lewis slipped from the room.

This was Ms. Acevedo's second baby and the delivery would be quick. She pushed with each contraction. Some of the baby's black hair was visible, slick with fluid. Between her pains I explained to the mother how we needed to clean the meconium out of her baby's mouth and nose before he started to cry. I alerted her that once the head came out she had to resist the powerful urge to push by blowing and panting, giving me a chance to suction the baby.

The head started to emerge. My fingers gently pressed on the back of the scalp, keeping the baby's chin tucked into its chest for an easier birth. First came the top of the head, then the forehead, eyebrows, nose, mouth and chin. Now came the time for the mother to pant. "Blow, blow, sople, sople," I urged her, manipulating one end of the suction tube into the baby's nostrils and then mouth, sucking on the other end. There is a natural pause in the birth process after the head comes out. From facing toward the mother's bottom the head does a half-turn to the left or right – external rotation is the medical term – before the shoulders deliver, The rest of the baby's body then slipped out quickly, along with a big gush of amniotic fluid.

"It's a boy, *varón*!" I announced, spitting out the suction tubing.

The pediatrician urged me to hurry, hurry. Firmly grasping the slippery, squirming infant between my left arm and my hip, my right hand reached for one clamp, then another. Once these are both clamped onto the umbilical cord it is safe to cut between them, separating mother and baby.

"Is he ok?" the mother asked. The baby answered her with a loud "wah, wah, wah," as the pediatrician whisked him away to the warm bassinet. With each cry the newborn inhaled more oxygen and his color became pinker. He waved his arms and kicked his legs. The Apgar score – based on a baby's cry, heart rate, color, reflexes and muscle tone – was a near-perfect 9 at one minute of life. He had not aspirated meconium.

"He is fine," the pediatrician assured Ms. Acevedo.

Finally a nurse arrived who knew the drill – how to take the baby's footprints and put on the hospital identity bracelets that link mother and baby.

Soon the mother felt another contraction and the placenta, or afterbirth, slid out. I massaged her abdomen to keep the uterus firm and prevent too much bleeding. All was well with the mother, she had not torn, needed no stitches. Then I carefully checked the placenta to be sure that it was complete and intact, with nothing left inside the patient to cause bleeding or infection.

"Want to see the afterbirth?" I offered. She was more interested in seeing her baby, now that the pediatrician was done examining him. The nurse put the tightly swaddled newborn in mama's arms. As she cuddled and whispered to her son I bathed the blood and amniotic fluid off her body with warm water.

When the patient was settled in the recovery room I looked for Mr. Lewis. He had finished his shift and gone home before I could thank him. He and I never discussed this incident afterwards. He could get fired for the good deed he had done. It was our secret.

Mr. and Mrs. Gomez

The white stretch limo idling in the semicircular driveway in front of Lincoln Hospital forced every eyeball to veer off course to check it out. People passing by inspected it – with open stares, sidewise glances, head-swiveling double-takes – and speculated about who the mystery visitor might be, perhaps some politician or rap star. This was the mid 1980s and stretch limousines were not common in Manhattan, let alone here in the Bronx.

I was on my way to the Chinese-Cuban restaurant across the street for lunch: rice with black beans, fried plaintains and café con leche, to go.

"No sugar," I reminded the thin man in a stained white apron behind the counter before he could dump three heaping teaspoons of it into the strong coffee.

"Bread?" he offered.

"Sure."

He threw several margarine-smeared hunks into the bag. Now I would be fortified for the next half of the 12-hour shift. I carried my lunch back to the hospital. The limo was still there.

Exiting the elevator and heading for Labor and Delivery to eat in the staff lounge, I saw Mr. Gomez pacing the hallway. His wife had given birth to a son two days before and it had been a pleasure to attend the birth. In their early thirties, married, planning the pregnancy, they seemed determined to raise their child in a world that had more to offer than the burned-out South Bronx of that time. He was a Vietnam veteran, working and going to college at night. Their love shone in the way she clung to him during labor and he quietly held her, cooling her face with a wet washcloth. In the delivery room he supported her head and whispered encouragement as she pushed. Some fathers position themselves at the foot of the delivery table to watch the baby emerge, yelling "push, push" from there. Mr. Gomez never left his wife's side until I asked if he wanted to cut the umbilical cord. I held his crying just-born son in my left arm, firmly braced against my body. With the other hand I held out the scissors, blade in my gloved hand, handle toward him. He seemed a bit tentative.

""Right there, between the clamps," I indicated the spot with the scissors. "Just don't touch me, my hands are sterile."

He cut.

"Here's your son," I said, placing the kicking baby in the bassinet for the nurse to take over: drying, foot-printing and putting on identity bands. I went back to the mother to deliver the afterbirth, monitor her bleeding and do suturing if necessary.

"You did a great job," I told her.

Behind me I could hear Vanessa, the nurse, congratulating Mr. Gomez. Soon she called out to me, "Apgar 9 at five minutes." When she finished her routines, Vanessa wrapped the baby tightly in blankets and brought him to Mrs. Gomez to hold. In his mother's arms, comforted by the swaddling and starting to adjust to the cold air and bright lights, the baby no longer cried. His parents beamed down at him.

Luckily that had been a quiet day in the maternity unit, so instead of rushing from patient to patient I could spend several hours with this couple during labor and do the delivery. Bonds between a woman, her family and midwife can form quickly in the intensity of labor and birth. The mother will remember her births as long as she lives, so in addition to providing safe care midwives try to make the experience as empowering as possible, an affirmation of the woman's strength.

Now, two days later, Mr. Gomez rushed over to me. He was wearing a white four-pocket guayabera shirt, a style popular in the Caribbean, and white pants.

"Please. Ellen," he said, "you have to help me."

"What's the matter," I asked, alarmed by the urgency in his voice and posture, "Is something wrong with the baby? Your wife?" My heart was beginning to gallop with fear.

"They're both fine," he said, "but I need the pediatrician to sign the baby's discharge papers right away." Walking as we talked we had now reached his wife's room. She too was dressed in white, her belly gently bulging under her blouse as if she were still 4 or 5 months pregnant. On the bed the baby's going home outfit and crocheted white blanket had been laid out.

"The newborn nursery told me they send the babies home at 10 a.m. but it's already nearly 1 p.m.," he fretted. "We've been waiting almost 3 hours."

"I'm sorry," I said, "They never finish the discharge paperwork before noon."

"Can't you talk to the pediatrician?" he asked. "Isn't there anything you can do to speed things up? I rented a limo to take my wife and baby home and the meter is running."

I am no fan of conspicuous displays, like gas-guzzling stretch limos, but Mr. Gomez's gesture of love for his wife and pride in his newborn child touched me deeply.

Dr. Khakoo

Dr. Khakoo's eggshell white pumps with two-inch heels tapped out her brisk pace. She even wore them in Labor and Delivery, covered with blue paper shoe covers when she did surgery. They were not shoes you would expect a woman in her fifties to wear while working on her feet all day.

Born in India, Dr. Khakoo adopted western clothing for work. In clinic she wore modest blouses and slacks, covered by a white lab coat with bulging pockets; in the delivery room she dressed, like everyone else, in blue scrub suits. Her dark hair was combed back from her face into a bun at the nape of her neck. As she went from patient to patient, hour after hour, little wisps escaped this proper hairdo, clinging to her forehead and cheeks. Small gold earrings glittered against her dark skin.

She drove a black Cadillac, never going faster than 40 miles an hour as other cars zipped past. We worked together at Lincoln and also in a prenatal clinic several miles from the hospital. She cared for high-risk patients while I saw women with uncomplicated pregnancies. When we finished examining patients at the same time – which did not happen often since she was much quicker than I was – Dr. Khakoo would offer to drive me back to the hospital. On one of those slow rides I told her how angry I felt at the way some of the male doctors treated our patients. I overheard one of them threaten a woman in labor that he would tell her husband how "badly" she behaved when she was in pain.

"They treat their wives and sisters the same way," Dr. Khakoo said in the low voice reserved for secrets and shameful things, looking straight ahead at the road.

One day she called me to her side in the gynecology clinic.

"Ellen, I am seeing a teenager and need a midwife consult." On the examining table was a 16-year-old with an enlarged spleen. The spleen is usually a fist-sized organ in the upper left part of the abdomen behind the rib cage. Viral infections such as mononucleosis and other diseases may cause it to swell to several times its normal size. With the patient's permission Dr. Khakoo guided my hands along the girl's left side. I could feel the spleen extend down to her hip bone. The doctor's request for a "consult" was her gentle way of teaching me something new.

Dr. Khakoo and the midwives formed a mutual admiration society.

"Mary Widhalm is a saint," she said whenever somebody mentioned our chief midwife.

Like her, we cared deeply about our patients and gave them all our energy and attention. She also understood and respected midwives. To her we were not just extra hands to help the doctors, but skilled practitioners with our own philosophy and holistic approach. She trusted us as the experts in normal pregnancy and birth, just as we relied upon her as the expert when complications arose.

I will never forget the day I watched Dr. Khakoo in action saving a baby's life. It was moderately busy in Labor and Delivery that Friday morning. Most of the six labor rooms were occupied but no other patients were lined up in stretchers in the hallway. When I helped Loretta, the patient in Labor Room 6, out of bed to go to the bathroom, her belly seemed huge. I read through her chart: she had been admitted by a very competent senior attending physician. He estimated this baby weighed eight pounds, the same size as her previous child.

The patient's labor had been progressing normally, then slowed down in the transition phase when the cervix goes from 8 to 10 centimeters dilated. Usually this phase, the most intense part of labor leading to a fully dilated cervix, lasts no more than one hour. When Loretta began to feel the urge to push I did a vaginal exam and found she was finally fully dilated after two hours in transition.

The mother pushed strongly with each contraction for an hour, the baby's head gradually coming down through her pelvis. As she got closer to giving birth I called in Dr. Hamid, the second-year obstetrics resident.

"This patient has gestational diabetes [diabetes of pregnancy], so she is high risk. A doctor should deliver her," I told him. I reviewed the information from the patient's prenatal chart with him, as well as the hospital admission note and the course of her labor. But did I share the nagging worry that this baby might be much bigger than the estimated 8 pounds?

Because this patient was diabetic we asked the pediatricians to be at the birth and wheeled Loretta to the delivery room. The nurse and I helped Loretta move from stretcher to delivery table, placing her legs in metal stirrups that held them wide apart. Under Dr. Hamid's fingers the baby's head slowly emerged. At this point during birth, the downward-facing head generally rotates 90 degrees to the left or right. Gently lowering the head between the attendant's hands will usually deliver the upper shoulder; then the rest of the body slides out.

This head did not budge. The doctor felt around the baby's neck to see if the umbilical cord was wrapped around it, impeding the birth. Nothing there.

"Shoulder dystocia!" Dr. Hamid said, "I need help." Shoulder dystocia is one of the most frightening childbirth emergencies. It occurs when the baby's head has emerged but the shoulders are stuck behind the pelvic bones and cannot be delivered with the usual maneuvers. The nurse and pediatrician helped Loretta pull her bent knees back against her abdomen, which usually will help deliver the shoulders, and urged her to push harder. A panicky atmosphere filled the room. We knew that the baby had to be delivered within minutes or suffer brain damage and possibly die.

I ran to get Dr. Khakoo, bursting into her office.

"Shoulder dystocia!" I said. She jumped up from her desk and followed me, her heels tapping urgently down the long corridor while I gave a panting summary of the situation.

Flinging open the delivery room door we saw the baby's body was still trapped inside the mother, and its head had turned an ugly blue color from lack of oxygen. Dr. Hamid was frantically trying to dislodge the shoulders and the pediatricians and nurses were yelling at the mother to push. I grabbed size seven sterile gloves and handed them to Dr. Khakoo. She pulled them on in an instant and elbowed the young doctor out of the way.

"Mother," she said to the patient, "this will hurt. Take a deep breath." She inserted her gloved right hand along the back of the baby's head and deep into Loretta's birth canal. Eyes closed, head bowed, the doctor planted her feet wide apart.

"Now push with all your strength," she commanded the patient. Dr. Khakoo leaned forward and performed some maneuver hidden inside the mother's body. The shoulder emerged slowly; the plump body followed, floppy as a rag doll. With a flash of instruments Dr. Khakoo clamped and cut the umbilical cord. A pediatrician snatched the baby boy in a towel and rushed him a few steps away to the warmed bassinet to begin resuscitation.

The baby did not cry or move. The first pediatrician covered the infant's face with a mask and pumped oxygen into his lungs. The other doctor pulled away the wet towel and rubbed a clean one over the motionless body, drying and stimulating. The baby's face was purplish blue, his body pale. His arms and legs were limp, the knees splayed out, but we saw his chest lift as each pump of oxygen expanded his lungs. Listening to the baby's chest with a stethoscope, the second pediatrician tapped out the too slow beat of the newborn's heart with his finger on the plastic bassinet so everyone could hear the rate. More than 100 beats a minute is a healthy pulse, but the doctor's finger was tapping more slowly.

"One minute," called the nurse timing the resuscitation.

"Is my baby all right?" asked the mother, lifting her head to watch what was going on. "Why isn't he crying?"

"The pediatrician is giving him oxygen with a mask over his face, so he cannot cry yet," Dr. Khakoo said. She snapped off the latex gloves. "Deliver the placenta," she told Dr. Hamid as she moved over to the bassinet.

The beat of the tapping finger was getter faster. The baby's arms and legs were starting to flex and move, no longer limp. He was becoming pinker. A thin cry came from under the mask, then a louder, stronger one. The chubby legs began to kick. One small fist waved. The pediatrician lifted the oxygen mask and the baby's now loud crying filled the room.

The doctors, nurses and I all exhaled with relief.

"Your baby needed some oxygen, but he sounds fine now," the pediatrician said over his shoulder to the mother, without taking his eyes off the baby.

"Five minutes," announced the nurse. "What's the Apgar score?"

"At one minute he had a slow heartbeat, but no spontaneous cry, bluish color and poor muscle tone, no reflex… Apgar one at one minute," said the pediatrician. An Apgar of one means a seriously oxygen-deprived baby that requires resuscitation.

"At five minutes he has a strong heartbeat and cry, good tone and reflexes," calculated the doctor. "Just one off for color," he said, looking at the baby's still slightly blue hands. "Apgar 9 at five minutes." A score of 7 or more indicates a vigorous newborn. This tough little boy went from motionless and not breathing to kicking and crying within minutes.

With the baby stable, the pediatrician began the routine newborn examination, from the fontanels or soft spots between the bones of his skull to the reflexes elicited by scratching the soles of his feet. On the right, the side where the shoulder had been wedged behind the mother's pubic bone, the baby was not moving his arm.

"Erb's palsy?" asked Dr. Khakoo softly.

The pediatrician nodded yes.

Erb's palsy occurs when nerves in the neck and shoulder are damaged, resulting in a weak or paralyzed arm. Fortunately more than nine out of ten such injuries will heal, either spontaneously or with physical therapy.

"How did you get the baby out?" I asked Dr. Khakoo as we left the delivery room, now that the emergency was over.

"He was getting limp from lack of oxygen. His shoulders were starting to slump. I just put some pressure on his back and that right shoulder slid under the mother's pubic bone," she said. "Let me know the baby's weight when they weigh him in the nursery. I pray the nerve damage heals," she added.

This was early in my career and my first experience with shoulder dystocia. I was relieved that I had turned the patient over to Dr. Hamid because the mother's diabetes made her high risk and not appropriate for a midwife delivery. But I felt guilty for failing to assess the size of the baby myself and just relying on someone else's notes, even though that person was a senior physician. I never repeated that mistake. The tape measure in my pocket might have warned me that the baby was much bigger than the 8 pounds estimated by the admitting doctor: the infant weighed 10 pounds 3 ounces.

Measuring abdomen size accurately is simple but vital. A belly more than 40 centimeters can indicate a potential problem: too much amniotic fluid, an extra-big baby or twins. We could have been more prepared – with Dr. Khakoo there from the beginning, rather than several precious minutes into the emergency, with the baby losing oxygen as each second ticked by and the nerves in the shoulder suffering damage from pressing against bone.

From that experience I learned to have confidence in what my hands and eyes told me. And above all to listen to the nagging worry or sudden sweat, as the body tries to warn of dangers that the mind has not yet organized into coherent thought.

In my purse I carried a list of maneuvers for dealing with shoulder dystocia. I reviewed it every single day of my working life before walking into Labor and Delivery. Over the years the paper became wrinkled and spotted with coffee stains. Making a xerox copy eliminated the wrinkles, but did not get rid of the stains. They just turned from coffee brown to ink black.

* * *

Dr. Khakoo died, only 68 years old, in 2004. Until I heard the Arabic name of the funeral parlor I did not realize that she belonged to the Muslim religious minority in predominantly Hindu India. Unsure what to expect at her funeral, I wore a scarf and clean socks, prepared to cover my head and take off my shoes, whatever was needed to show respect. Mary and I traveled together by subway to the service. Behind corrugated steel gates in post-9/11 Queens, the one-storey madrassa in which the funeral took place vibrated slightly to the roar of low-flying jets taking off and landing at nearby JFK Airport.

A chartered bus brought scores of co-workers from the hospital where she had cared for patients until just hours before her death.

"She was tired when she came home that evening," her husband told mourners. She went to bed and died of a heart attack before dawn. It was just like Dr. Khakoo, everybody agreed, to keep working until the very end.

Dr. Khakoo's body was covered by a simple white shroud. Only females were allowed to view the corpse. The men gathered in a separate room; a small loudspeaker on the wall carried the sound of prayers from their section to ours. While most of us sat on the floor a dozen women performed ritual motions, alternately standing, kneeling and touching their foreheads to the ground, wrapping and unwrapping their headscarves in a somber dance of farewell.

Mrs. Roberts

Dr. Morgan flung open the swinging doors to Labor and Delivery.

"Here's one for you, Ellen," he said, indicating the hugely pregnant woman clinging to the side rails of a stretcher. I greeted the patient and wheeled her into the first empty labor room on the long corridor that led to the delivery and operating suites.

The doctor's admission note stated that Mrs. Roberts was a 37-year old woman who had four previous vaginal births without complications, but no prenatal care with the current pregnancy. He measured her abdomen at 40 centimeters, the right size for a full-term pregnancy. She was in active labor – her cervix was 5 centimeters (out of 10) dilated – and the baby was in vertex (head first) position. By Dr. Morgan's estimate the baby weighed about 7 ½ pounds. The fetal heart was beating 144 times a minute. These were all normal findings

A woman who has had other babies often goes rapidly from 5 centimeters to fully dilated and ready to deliver, so I quickly did my own assessment. Experience had taught me to thoroughly examine every patient and not simply rely on what other people wrote. Between contractions Mrs. Roberts told me that, after all those other pregnancies, "I know the drill," and did not bother with prenatal clinic. "And I don't smoke or do drugs, pregnant or not," she said.

Mrs. Roberts was a big woman, but fat alone could not account for the 45 centimeter abdomen that I measured – off the charts in terms of size. Examining her belly, I felt the baby's head down by the mother's pubic bone. Vertex presentation, as Dr. Morgan had noted. Near the top of her abdomen I could feel the soft roundness of the baby's buttocks. But what were these other lumps and bumps?

"Mrs. Roberts," I asked, "Does anyone in your family have twins?"

"Yeah," she said, "me. My eight-year-old daughters are twins." There was no mention of that in the chart. Was Dr. Morgan too preoccupied with the love of his life, the first model of the new Lexus luxury car, to notice these little details?

"How does this belly feel?" I was still trying to figure out exactly what my fingers were touching, but almost certain there was more than one baby.

"Big," she said, "Lots of kicking… You think it's twins?" She seemed to take this possibility calmly.

I put the fetal monitor below her navel to listen to the heart tones of the head-first baby, placing my stethoscope in different positions to try and pick up a second heartbeat. I could hear something, but it was not different enough from the beat on the monitor to be sure it was another baby. A strong contraction made me stop. The patient was getting more uncomfortable – and closer to giving birth – with each one.

"We need a sonogram to be sure," I said. "I'm going to get the doctor. Remember, my name is Ellen. Scream for me as loud as you can if you feel the baby coming."

"You know I will," she said.

I ran to the staff lounge and grabbed Dr. Clark, one of my favorite attending physicians. He respected the midwives' judgment and vice versa. In a crisis he always remained calm, in control. When we needed help he responded immediately, not making us go through the chain of command by first consulting the inexperienced second-year resident.

"It must be another set of twins," I said, concluding a quick summary of the case.

"Troublemaker," he said to me, wheeling the portable sonogram machine into the patient's room. The image on the screen revealed a second fetus, its head partly hidden behind the chest of baby number one, also in vertex position.

"You know what this means?" he asked Mrs. Roberts.

"Double trouble," she said, pointing her chin at me. "The midwife already told me." She was starting to breathe hard with another contraction.

"You need a C-section," Dr. Clark told her.

"No way, doc!" she said. "I had my other twins natural. I can do it again. Don't cut me open."

"Vertex, vertex," I said quietly, meaning that with both babies coming head first the chances for a safe vaginal birth were excellent.

Another, stronger, contraction came and went. Dr. Clark did a pelvic exam. "Your cervix is fully dilated," he said to the patient. "We're going to the delivery room right now. You need to push with everything you've got if you don't want a C-section."

"I can do it," Mrs. Roberts said.

Dr. Clark must have also been thinking that with both babies in the right position, the mother's history of delivering twins normally – and her desire to do so now – that vaginal birth was a safer option. Surgery always has the potential for bleeding and infection. Given Mrs. Robert's age, African-American race and excess weight, an immediate Cesarean section under general anesthesia greatly increased the risk of complications for the mother. A blood clot that could travel to her lungs or brain and fatally cut off circulation to those organs was at the top of the list of dangers.

Dr. Clark started wheeling her stretcher down the hall. I ran to the nurses' station to alert Head Nurse Perez to have the delivery room set up for twins. She told the ward clerk to page the anesthesiologist and pediatrician right away. We called anesthesia "just in case" and pediatricians were routinely called for the birth of twins, who are often born prematurely, as well as for patients who had no prenatal care.

When I returned to the delivery room Mrs. Roberts was on the table and Dr. Clark had scrubbed in. The nurses had brought an extra bassinet and were filling out ID bands for 'Roberts, baby A' and 'Roberts, baby B.' The mother pushed like a champ, and Dr. Clark caught baby A, a full-term girl who cried immediately and pinked up nicely from the oxygen she inhaled. He cut the cord and the pediatrician took the infant to the bassinet.

Now came the tricky part: delivering the second twin. Dr. Clark snapped off his gloves and guided the ultrasound probe over Mrs. Roberts' only slightly deflated abdomen. "We're OK," he said, "twin B is still vertex." He moved the probe higher, until it located the baby's heart. On the screen we could see it contracting with each beat. "Ellen, hold this so we can monitor the heartbeat." I took the probe and kept one eye on the screen. The heart continued contracting rhythmically.

Dr. Clark put a new pair of size 8 ½ sterile gloves on his big hands. "Mommy," he said to the patient, "You have to do exactly what I tell you."

"Sure, doc," she said. "Tell me when to push."

The doctor did another vaginal exam. "Amni hook," he said. His right hand still inside the mother, Dr. Clark held up his left hand to receive the sterile instrument used to break the membranes around baby B. This was good news. It meant the second baby was in its own sac of amniotic fluid, and the head was deep enough in the mother's pelvis to safely rupture the membranes. The nurse put the amni hook in his hand.

"Ready?" he asked Mrs. Roberts.

"Should I push now?" she said.

"Not until I tell you." Dr. Clark slid the instrument inside her. His left hand twisted as he maneuvered the handle to grasp the membranes with the small metal hook, then withdrew it as half a cup of clear fluid gushed out.

"Now, push!" he ordered. Mrs. Roberts gave a deep grunting push. "Stop," he said as the contraction ebbed. A few contractions and pushes later twin B, a boy, was born. He was as vigorous as his minutes-older sister.

The mother lay back on the table, exhausted and relieved. "I told you I could do it," she said to the doctor.

A birth is not complete when the baby is born. The third stage of labor then begins, and only ends with the delivery of the placenta. With twins the uterus is much more distended, making it more difficult for that organ to contract. This contraction is what expels the afterbirth and then seals off the open blood vessels in the uterine wall where the placenta or placentas had been implanted. Hemorrhage is a danger if the uterus does not contract properly.

"Is the Pit ready?" Dr. Clark asked the circulating nurse. Pitocin is a drug that makes the uterus contract and is used to prevent or treat postpartum hemorrhage. "Push 30 units in the IV bag the instant the placentas are out."

"Right here," she said, holding up the syringe.

There were two placentas and they both delivered without problem. Pitocin and massaging the abdomen helped the uterus contract firmly. There was no hemorrhage. Healthy mother, two healthy babies, weighing a total of almost 14 pounds. Everything was good.

And I had a great story to tell my family and friends.

Lissette

Lissette was 18 years old when she started prenatal care. A first prenatal visit is a comprehensive examination which includes taking a history of the patient's health throughout her life, the current and any prior pregnancies, doing a head to toe physical exam, including a pelvic exam, Pap smear and tests for sexually transmitted infections. A crucial component is to assign a due date, based on her last menstrual period (hopefully she remembers) and the size of her uterus on physical exam. Sonograms were reserved for problem cases, not routinely done then. Patients were asked about smoking, drinking and drugs. We try to establish a human connection as we talk with and examine the patient. We are allotted 30 minutes to accomplish all this plus do the paperwork.

The pregnancy, her first, was not planned but Lissette said she was happy to be having a baby. She was a pretty, dark-haired teenager who answered all my questions eagerly, got undressed and into a cloth gown and hopped onto the examining table. Head, neck, heart, lungs, breasts – all normal. By her last period she was 14 weeks pregnant, a little more than three months. On abdominal exam I felt the top of her uterus just above the pubic bone, the size confirming the due date.

"Your baby should be born September 22, give or take two weeks," I said. "Remember, it's an estimate, not a guarantee." It was too early to hear the baby's heartbeat with my fetoscope – a stethoscope with a large trumpet-shaped bell for picking up fetal heart tones around five months.

Then it was time for the speculum exam. A speculum is a metal or plastic instrument that is inserted into the vagina and then opened to hold the walls of the vagina apart so the cervix, or mouth of the womb, can be visualized to do a Pap or other test. Most women find it uncomfortable or embarrassing. Many do not hesitate to tell me so. A common gesture is to close or cover her eyes, as if not looking will make the unpleasant situation disappear. Or as if closing her eyes will somehow prevent me from seeing the hidden part of her body that too many women are taught to be ashamed of.

"Please move your bottom down to the end of the table," I said, "and put your feet into the stirrups." The glass slides for the Pap smear and culture plate for gonorrhea testing were all laid out, along with the speculum and cue tips for taking the specimens. Before putting on sterile latex gloves I helped patients get into position. But Lissette clamped her bent knees together and covered her face with both hands. Her breathing was ragged, fighting sobs. I was about to tell her to relax, let your knees drop apart and breathe slowly – the usual not terribly helpful instructions. But my body rather than my mind sensed her special fear and heard the message she was silently screaming.

"Lissette," I asked softly, "did anybody ever hurt you down there?" She gave a tiny nod, yes, from behind her hands.

"I'm so sorry… It was not your fault," I said, struggling to figure out how to handle this situation.

Then, "I'm not going to do the vaginal exam. Please sit up." She sat up. Her hands came away from her face, but her eyes stayed fixed on her knees. I can only begin to imagine how hard this was for her.

"You will be coming to see me for the next six months," I said. "When we know each other better, when you feel you can trust me, when you are ready for me to examine you, let me know. OK? We don't have to do it today. I'm not even going to mention it again. I'll wait until you tell me." She gave a tiny nod of agreement.

"But there is one thing I have to do," I added. "I have to send you to the social worker to talk about what happened to you and how to keep you safe from the person who hurt you." Another tiny nod.

"It's not my baby's father," she said, barely above a whisper. "He's nice to me."

"I'm glad to hear that," I said. "You can get dressed now."

My 1977 edition of Danforth's *Obstetrics and Gynecology*, a major textbook that we studied in midwifery school, makes no mention of sexual abuse. It devotes one page to rape – when recognized as such and reported to authorities by an adult. It was not until 1989 that New York State passed legislation requiring health care workers and teachers to be trained to recognize and report child abuse. Social workers and other therapists were included under the law only years later.

This encounter with Lissette was not the first time I cared for a patient who had been sexually abused, either as a child or as a woman. Some had been able to speak to me about it or perhaps had come to terms with their fear of vaginal exams. Lissette had no words to describe what she had experienced; she could only curl up in the fetal position and hide her face. Surely there had been others who I failed to recognize, too meek, ashamed or frightened to give the least hint of the abuse they had suffered, too fearful to resist or complain about my well-intentioned probing.

I have tried hard to recall Lissette's visits with me for the rest of her pregnancy. My memory is a complete blank. The only explanation I can think of is that those other visits were completely routine, nothing special to stick in my mind. It must mean that, at some point in the following months, she said, "I'm ready."

Thank you, Lissette, for reminding me about listening to patients, whether they use words or silence or speak with their body, and no matter how painful the message she struggles to communicate. How brave you were to come to prenatal clinic, wanting to take good care of your baby in spite of the examination that terrified you.

Personal best

My husband and I were meeting friends at a Greenwich Village restaurant for a late dinner after my 12-hour labor room shift. Sitting at the bar nibbling pretzels while waiting for the other couple to arrive I described a busy and fulfilling day at work. After listening to my story John waved the bartender over.

"Give this lady a drink," he said, pride in his voice. "She delivered five babies today." When the bartender looked puzzled, my husband clarified, "Five babies of five other women." I probably ordered a glass of white wine, or maybe just ginger ale. I was already high from the wonder and adrenalin rush of birth – and of being able to perform at my peak as a confident midwife with nearly six years of experience.

Although I cannot recall the details of those five births, I will never forget the feeling of days like that in Lincoln's labor room. Delivering babies puts you at the pulsating core of life. The sound of the fetal heartbeat is the ever-present background music. It is a privilege to help women go through the experience of childbearing, each in her own way. The patient may call on Jesus, Allah or mama (mama being by far the most frequent choice) but I am the one with the awesome responsibility of caring for mother and babe. Fortunately, nature has stacked the deck in our favor: the vast majority of births are normal and uncomplicated.

On those hectic days I could not always remember every patient's name. "Mommy," I would address those who spoke English, "mi hija" (my daughter) for the Spanish speakers. In my mind I visualized the six labor rooms and the other women on stretchers in the hallway, keeping track of how far along in labor each one was, trying to estimate when they would deliver, alert to any potential problems.

Should I try to hasten a birth by breaking the bag of water around the fetus? Was it a good time to give a mother a narcotic for pain relief, or would that cause her baby to be born too sleepy? I was a general in command of a one-woman army, carefully planning my strategy and tactics. The enemy was lack of time to spend comforting and supporting each laboring patient. And forget about taking a few minutes for something to eat or a sip of water; I could barely manage a bathroom break.

With parched lips, damp armpits and hair shoved under a blue paper shower cap I was not the well-groomed professional you see on a television hospital show. A surgical mask from the previous delivery might hang around my neck like a bib; the mask's plastic edge leaving reddened indentations across my nose and cheeks. The pockets of my lab coat and scrub pants bulged with supplies, including several pairs of sterile gloves in case they were needed immediately with no time to run to the supply cabinet as a baby started to emerge. There were also scraps of paper on which I scribbled the name, sex, time of birth and Apgar score of each baby I delivered: these were needed for notes in the medical record and to fill out birth certificates when I got a free moment to do the paperwork.

Attending five births in one day was a record for me. But it could not top the six deliveries my co-worker Sister Maureen had done in a single shift. She also held the impossible-to-beat record for delivering two babies at the same time. Both mothers were ready to give birth simultaneously but there was only one person available to attend them. Luckily that one person was this resourceful midwife. Nurses put the women on stretchers side by side in the same delivery room and kept handing Sister Maureen fresh pairs of sterile gloves as she caught baby # 1 then changed gloves to catch baby # 2. With a new pair of clean gloves she went back to mom # 1 for the placenta and repeated the same move for the second lady's placenta.

On another occasion Sister Maureen had answered the urgent call "the baby is coming" – or maybe it was Mr. Lewis saying "come quick, Sister," – to deliver a woman in the elevator.

Ms. James

Ms. James was in family planning clinic for a routine "pill check" visit. This was scheduled about ten weeks after a patient received her first three-month supply of birth control pills. The midwife would check for any troublesome side effects and, if the patient was satisfied with this method, give her another six-month or one-year supply. I had never met Ms. James before, so I reviewed her medical record before calling her into my room, noting that the Pap test done at the previous visit showed some non-specific inflammation and that she had lost 10 pounds since then. Her blood pressure today was normal. She was a neatly groomed 31-year-old black woman, a non-smoker, slightly overweight but certainly not obese. She had no history of medical problems.

"How do you like these birth control pills?" I asked, after introducing myself and seating her on the examining table.

"Actually, I never started taking them," she said. "I'm not having sex, so why bother." Then she added, "The nurse told me there was a problem with my Pap test. What's wrong?"

"Just some inflammation," I said. "It's not cancer, not a sexually transmitted disease. We'll give you a vaginal cream to use for a week. That should clear it up."

"Thank God," she said. "I was scared it was something serious."

"Come back in six months and we'll repeat the Pap test," I said while writing an order for the cream. Everything required according to the protocol for a pill check follow-up was done. I could have ushered Ms. James out to pick up the medication and make her next appointment. But I remembered the weight loss and asked, "You lost 10 pounds since the last visit. Are you on a diet?"

"No," she said.

"Any reason to be losing weight? No appetite? Anything worrying you?" I probed.

"Well… " said Ms. James, "I heard an old boyfriend of mine died a while back. That was upsetting news…" Pause. "And I get out of breath going up the stairs to my apartment."

"How many flights is it?" I said.

"Second floor," she answered.

"Let me listen to your lungs," I said, putting my stethoscope in my ears. She lifted her blouse and I put the bell on her chest. "Take a deep breath with your mouth wide open." I could hear her inhale through her mouth but no sound came from the stethoscope. "Again." Still no sound. I put the stethoscope on her back. "Deep breath." Still no sound of air moving into her lungs. I was worried that this could be pneumonia, and about to get one of the physicians to check my findings, when Ms. James said, "By the way, what is this?" pointing to her mouth.

Experience had taught me that "by the way" was often followed by the question the patient most wanted – and most feared – to ask. Sometimes it was only with her hand on the door knob, about to leave the examining room, that she got up the courage to ask, knowing that it was now or never.

She opened her mouth wide. The throat, tongue and mucous membrane lining the insides of her cheeks were covered with the white, cheesy coating of a yeast infection. This kind of thrush is fairly common in babies, but only seen in adults when the immune system is not functioning. The pieces of the puzzle all began to fit together. Weight loss, pneumonia, oral thrush, the minor inflammation on the Pap test, the dead boyfriend: Ms. James had AIDS.

My stomach knotted and my brain went blank trying to figure out what to say. How do you tell a woman she has AIDS? In 1989 many people still thought AIDS was strictly a disease of gay men and injection drug users. It was a fatal disease with an inexorable course of wasting and succumbing to infections that an intact immune system could easily fight off; powerful medications to combat the virus would not be developed until years later. Did my face give away the thoughts racing through my mind? Could she smell my sweaty anxiety?

Then Ms. James made it easy for me. "Will people discriminate against me if I have HIV?" she said. She already knew.

I took the stethoscope out of my ears and wrapped it around my neck. I can't remember if I put a comforting hand on her arm as a gesture to show I was not afraid to touch her, or tried to regain my composure with a more formal and distant posture.

"It is illegal to discriminate against HIV-positive people," was the best I could do. "And everything in this clinic is confidential." But we both understood such laws were a feeble defense against gossip or the rampant fear and hatred of people with the AIDS virus, and those perceived as being at high risk of having HIV. I suggested she go to a clinic that specialized in treating HIV-positive women.

"I know too many people who work at that hospital," she said, worried they might learn about her diagnosis. She left weighing the options of going to a respected North Bronx hospital or to the Gay Men's Health Crisis clinic for testing, referral and support. GMHC describes itself as "the world's first and leading provider of HIV/AIDS prevention, care and advocacy." It was formed by activists in 1981 when the medical profession, public health officials and even many in the gay community were all reluctant to respond to the looming AIDS crisis.

Ms. James' path crossed mine for the first and last time that day. Looking back on our encounter I wonder whether I did her a service by confirming her worst fear at a time when effective treatment was not yet available. She already had multiple signs and symptoms of a damaged immune system. I doubt if she survived long enough to be helped by the new generations of powerful anti-HIV medications that would be developed starting in 1996.

A few years later I would be hired by the Center for Mother and Baby Care, the clinic specializing in treating HIV-positive women and their children, the clinic I had suggested Ms. James attend.

Shaniqua

Shaniqua had attended childbirth preparation classes in Teen Clinic so she knew better than to rush to the hospital when the cramps of early labor woke her that morning. She waited until the contractions came every five minutes – strong enough to make her clutch her boyfriend's shoulders – before coming to Labor and Delivery. In the triage room she pouted when I said that the midwife who had cared for her at every check-up in Teen Prenatal Clinic was not on duty that day. She would have to make do with me.

"At least you're a lady," she consoled herself. The good news for Shaniqua was that she was already 6 centimeters (out of 10) dilated, in active labor.

"How much longer..." she started to ask when another contraction interrupted the question. She leaned forward, left hand braced against left thigh, right hand rubbing the bottom of her belly. My hands rubbed low on her back until the pain ebbed.

"You're going fast. Another hour or so and you'll be ready to push this baby out," I said. "Pushing is a big relief from these pains. Let's get you into a labor room."

The six labor rooms were full, so my patient climbed onto a stretcher in Labor Room 1 where another woman occupied the bed. Ms. Perez, the head nurse, planted her 4 foot 11 inch body in the doorway to bar Shaniqua's boyfriend Mike from entering the room.

"But we went to childbirth classes," he pleaded, pulling out a wrinkled Certificate of Completion to prove it.

Ms. Perez was unmoved. "There's another patient in that room. How would you like it if her man was in there looking up between your girlfriend's legs?"

"I don't want to look at nothing but Shaniqua," he said, "and she wants me there. I promised I wouldn't leave her."

But this was Perez's domain and the so-called hospital rules were her way of running the place, no exceptions allowed.

"You want me to call security?" she said. New York City's municipal hospital system has its own police, a 1,000-plus person force half-way between minimum-wage security guards and NYPD officers.

Before this escalated further I took Mike aside. "Soon as she has her own room or we go to the delivery room I will come get you," I promised. "Don't leave the waiting area. I'll explain to Shaniqua why you can't be with her." He had no choice but to comply.

Two other patients needed my care, and as I was charting my notes I heard Shaniqua's panicky cry: "The baby is coming!"

Those words must never be ignored. I ran to her room. The baby certainly was coming, the fluffy-haired head almost halfway out.

"Don't push, blow, blow!" I commanded. No time to put on the gloves I always carried in my pocket. Shaniqua was yelling and the patient in the other bed was staring and I was shouting "Delivery in Room 1" hoping for assistance. And then the baby was in my bare hands crying "wah, wah, wah" at the top of her lungs and Shaniqua was laughing instead of yelling. Amniotic fluid that gushed out with the baby soaked through my scrubs down to my underwear. I searched for a dry piece of sheet to cover the baby. I put her on her mother's chest and proclaimed "Girl!" Shaniqua was cooing, "My baby, my baby, my beautiful baby," as she held the wet, wailing newborn in her arms. The other lady in the room shook her head saying, "Damn, girl, I've been here for hours and you're done ahead of me."

The nurse came flying in with a blue rubber bulb syringe to suction out the baby's nose and mouth, but this little girl didn't need any help with her breathing. She already had the lovely rose sepia color of black babies when they are first born and full of oxygen, before they turn their proper darker shade of brown. The nurse handed me a basin with sterile clamps and a scissor to cut the cord. But one of my tricks was to wait to cut the cord so nobody could snatch the still-attached baby away from its mother. The baby also receives more blood and oxygen from the placenta via an uncut umbilical cord, not that this little Amazon needed it.

"Thanks, Ms. Wright." I said to the nurse. "Please get the father from the waiting room. His name is Mike. I'll bring mommy and baby to the delivery room. You and daddy can meet us there."

The other reason I did not cut the umbilical cord is that I had inadvertently lied to Mike when I promised to get him for the delivery, so I wanted to console him by offering to let him cut the cord. Fathers usually loved that – if they were not too afraid of messing it up.

"It's like cutting a fingernail: it doesn't hurt," I would reassure them.

I pushed the stretcher down the long corridor. It was a pretty easy one-person job, not heavy and bulky like a regular hospital bed, but Mr. Hernandez, the housekeeper, helped me and congratulated the mother while we moved her and the baby into the delivery room.

Ms. Wright brought Mike after getting him properly suited up in scrubs, cap, mask and shoe covers, maintaining the fiction that some sterile process was going on here. Now Shaniqua was feeling great and bubbling proudly over how the baby came out so fast, "mostly before the midwife got there." Mike cut the cord without hesitation and accepted my apology and excuse – "I just barely got there myself" – for not calling him in time for the birth. Mommy and daddy had a brief moment to marvel at their daughter; then hospital protocol took over as the nurse footprinted the baby and put on her wrist and ankle identity bands. Bonding and breastfeeding were tolerated, but never took priority over rules and routines.

The placenta delivered as easily as the baby, but with considerably less drama. Not much blood was lost and no stitches were needed. Ms. Wright brought a clean, dry stretcher and we helped Shaniqua onto it.

"Say bye bye for now," the nurse told the young parents, presenting the baby, now expertly swaddled, for them to kiss.

"How much does she weigh?" asked Shaniqua. That is usually the first question mothers ask once they know their baby's sex.

"She'll get weighed in the newborn nursery," Ms. Wright said. Hefting the baby in her experienced hands she added, "My guess is 7 pounds. Good job."

Will you be there?

"Will you be with me when I have my baby?" patients asked me as their due date neared.

"Yes," I said, "If you go into labor on a Friday." That was my assigned day to work in Lincoln's labor room. Continuity of care

– meaning one person caring for a woman throughout pregnancy and birth – is a cherished midwife ideal. It is possible in a small practice with a few births each month. In a busy city hospital where I saw more than 30 prenatal patients every week it was not often possible. My schedule was fixed, but it could not hurt to plant the idea of giving birth on a Friday in the women's minds.

Ms. Ahmed had a special reason to ask if I would deliver her baby; her Muslim religion called for women to be attended only by women in childbirth.

"Other midwives work in the labor room, and there are female doctors," I said. "But try to have your baby on Friday, with me."

Ms. Ahmed did not cover her black wavy hair. Wearing the traditional Pakistani shalwar kameez – a long tunic over loose pants – she did not look properly dressed for the harsh Bronx winter. But rolling down the pants to examine her pregnant belly, I saw the waffle-weave men's long underwear that kept her warm beneath the bright orange outfit of light cotton. The pale stretch marks on her abdomen testified that this was her third or fourth child. Now in the ninth month of pregnancy she was scheduled for weekly clinic visits. As she left each check-up I reminded her, "We have a date on Friday."

It was late into my 12-hour labor room stint – the 4 p.m. shift of nurses was already on duty – when Ms. Ahmed arrived. The joy at seeing each other was mutual.

"I didn't think you would still be here," she said, between the strong contractions that made her clutch my arm.

"I work until 8 o'clock," I said. "We've got plenty of time." My vaginal exam found her to be 7 centimeters dilated. Barely an hour later, I caught her daughter.

Women usually bond quickly with a midwife in labor, even if they have not had any previous relationship. But continuity of care is so much better.

* * *

My other Friday date was with my husband, who had a big pot of pasta ready when I got home, ravenous, around 9 o'clock. We ate and then watched "Miami Vice," a cop show whose run coincided with my years working in the Bronx. Its lush sets, pounding soundtrack and high-energy violence helped me wind down after work. Compared to a long day in Labor and Delivery at Lincoln "Miami Vice" seemed relaxing.

The Happy Land fire

My Arthur Avenue clinic was not far from the Happy Land social club where a fire killed 87 people, mostly immigrants from Honduras, on March 25, 1990. This was exactly 79 years after the Triangle Shirtwaist Fire in lower Manhattan killed 146 mainly young Jewish and Italian women garment factory workers. Several of my patients were Honduran and I dreaded hearing that one of them had died in such a horrible way.

Later that year I began to look for another job. I loved my sister midwives at Lincoln. We were a great team made up of very different individuals, all deeply committed to our patients and supportive of each other. Sister Maureen and Mary had given me quiet emotional support through the many crises of my son's ongoing illness. I liked and respected several of the doctors, even when we did not share the same philosophy about birth. But for some reason the Happy Land tragedy broke my spirit. I just could not go on working in this devastated landscape.

St Luke's/Roosevelt Hospital, 1990–91

Going from Lincoln to St. Luke's/Roosevelt was a big change. My new workplace was a private non-profit Manhattan hospital network that also accepted Medicaid. Although the clinic patients were similar to those in the Bronx, and there was an evening Teen Clinic, the location and resources were worlds apart with more staff, better equipment and higher pay. The Roosevelt division in midtown mainly served privately-insured patients, including those of a well-established midwifery service. The St. Luke's division was across from Columbia University; it was lovely to walk through the leafy campus rather than gritty Bronx streets on my way to and from work..

At Roosevelt a large health maintenance organization provided maternity care for members of several unions, religious groups, city workers and people on staff at the United Nations. Their clients were private patients but were managed by the residents as well as by physicians from the HMO. As a staff midwife I also took care of these patients. They ran the gamut from teachers and transit workers to Orthodox Jewish 'grand multiparas' (mothers having borne five or more children), UN personnel from around the world and members of the Unification Church, a religious group pejoratively called 'Moonies,' who lived in the New Yorker Hotel not far from the hospital.

Mrs. Levine

Mrs. Levine was in labor with her second baby. She was part of an Orthodox Jewish community in Brooklyn whose members married young and bore many children. At 24 she only had one child while friends and relatives the same age already had several. She was glad to have me attend her rather than the male obstetrician from her HMO.

Men of her religion do not touch their wives during labor or view the birth. Her husband was elsewhere, praying for a safe delivery. Her mother-in-law sat at the bedside and another relative cared for Ms. Levine's 3-year old daughter. That little girl, Chava, had been born very prematurely, weighing just two pounds and a few ounces. Women who have one premature birth are at risk of early delivery with subsequent babies; fortunately this current pregnancy had gone to term.

"Chava was in intensive care for a long time," Mrs. Levine told me as she labored. "We did not know if she was going to live or die. I pumped my milk, but she was too weak to suck from a bottle. They had to feed her through a tube. She was in Beth Israel Hospital in Manhattan and every day my husband and I traveled from Brooklyn to be with her. Then came Pesach." Pesach or Passover is the eight-day spring holiday celebrating the Jews' escape from slavery in Egypt.

"We are not allowed to travel by car or subway during Pesach. But I could feel my baby needed me. I told my husband, 'we are walking to see Chava.' And we did, all the way from Brooklyn, over the bridge, to the hospital. When we got to intensive care the baby heard my voice and turned her little head to look at me. That was when I knew my daughter would live."

Mrs. Levine paused intermittently during this story, breathing through contractions, her eyes closed. Deep into her body, she did not moan or cry. I felt unsure if rubbing her back or her feet would be received as comforting or intrusive. I stood at her side with my hands in my pockets, murmuring encouragement and glancing from time to time at the monitor showing a regular fetal heartbeat. She was in the most intense stage of labor.

A few contractions later, "I need to push," she said urgently. My vaginal exam confirmed that she was ready. The nurse prepared the betadine wash for cleaning the mother and the instruments for clamping and cutting the umbilical cord while I scrubbed my hands at the sink. The rooms in this hospital were used for labor, birth and recovery afterwards. It was much better for the patient. Forcing a woman to move from the labor bed onto a stretcher – to be pushed to a delivery/operating room – and then move from the stretcher to the delivery table was miserable.

"What? You want me to move now!?" many a mother balked at being ordered to perform these acrobatics in the moments just before her baby was born.

"Please don't cut an episiotomy," Mrs. Levine said as I put on sterile gloves.

"I don't plan to," I told her. "Just listen when I tell you to stop pushing and pant as the baby comes out." When the vagina stretches slowly with gentle pushing there is less chance that the mother will tear.

"Would you like to deliver lying on your side?" I said. Some mothers were more comfortable in that position. With knees bent, one leg on the bed and the other slightly elevated with the foot resting on my hip, this side-lying position did not require a woman to spread her legs wide apart. When preserving modesty might be a concern for the mother I offered this option.

"No!" Mrs. Levine rejected the idea, choosing the half-sitting position always shown in television births. The nurse elevated the patient's head and placed her legs in metal stirrups that attached to the bed. With little grunts and puffs she pushed her baby into my hands fifteen minutes later.

"A boy!" I put him directly on his mother's abdomen and he started crying immediately. The nurse dried him with a warm towel while Mrs. Levine enfolded her son in her arms and spoke words I could not understand. The mother-in-law, who had kept silently in the background, now stepped in close to look at her healthy grandson, smiling and crying at the same time and patting the mother's shoulder.

"Mazel tov," I said. That was about the extent of my Yiddish, a language my grandparents and parents spoke when they did not want the children to understand what was being said, and never taught to me or my siblings.

I cut the cord so Mrs. Levine could put the baby to her breast while he was in the active alert stage right after birth. With a bit of help the newborn found the nipple; his mother gave a deep sigh as he latched on and began to suck. Nursing helped the placenta deliver; there was just a small gush of blood.

After the long anxious months she had been through with her premature daughter, it was lovely for me to be able to put a healthy full term baby in Mrs. Levine's arms. The little boy weighed almost seven pounds and went home with his parents on his second day of life, joining the big sister who almost had not survived.

Marlene

The clerks who made up the clinic schedule assigned deaf patients to me. I had attended sign language classes at my local Y and although my signing skills were minimal and I always tried to arrange for a sign language interpreter to be present I welcomed the chance to practice and enjoyed working with deaf patients. Marlene was one of them.

She was young and healthy; her pregnancy was uncomplicated. As her due date approached I gave her my beeper number and a note requesting that Labor and Delivery personnel contact me when she was admitted. I was a staff midwife with a fixed schedule in the prenatal clinic but nobody cared which hours I worked on Labor and Delivery as long as I put in my time. Each month I picked a few favorite patients who would be delivering soon and told them to page me when they were admitted in labor so that I – rather than the resident on duty – could attend their birth. I could not promise to always be available, but I would try.

My patients were too considerate: they never woke me at 3 a.m. or even called after midnight. One woman was admitted around 10 p.m.

"My husband said it was too late to call," she told me when I visited her on the postpartum unit the next day and asked why she had not paged me. How disappointed I felt to miss this birth. Her baby had been born just after 1 a.m. – a short stint on a midwife's clock.

Marlene went into labor in the early evening. One of the nurses paged me and I was at the hospital 15 minutes later, since I lived less than two miles away. Marlene paced in her room – staying upright and in motion helps the baby descend in the pelvis and stimulates contractions. She felt better walking than lying in bed. We monitored the baby's heartbeat with a belt around her abdomen and were reassured by a pattern of about 140 beats per minute that periodically sped up to 160. The length of the wires that ran to the machine limited how far she could go – back and forth, a radius of less than three feet in a semi-circle in front of the monitor. She never complained or indicated she was in pain. Perhaps deafness had insulated her from the scare stories about birth that people inflict on pregnant women. I had noticed a similar calm reaction to labor in others also isolated from the culture of fear, such as women with severe psychiatric problems or developmental delay.

By 10 p.m. Marlene was in advanced labor, 7 centimeters dilated. But then her labor stalled. At midnight she was still the same. Feeling the fontanels, or soft spots between the bones of the baby's head, my vaginal exam revealed that its position was occiput posterior, meaning the back of its skull was towards the mother's back rather than on one side or towards the front. The posterior position makes birth more difficult, and sometimes impossible.

From my midwife bag of tricks we tried various postures that usually help facilitate birth. Marlene labored on her side and then on hands and knees, but neither caused the baby to rotate into a better position. We tried modern medicine too: Pitocin strengthened the contractions, but failed to dilate her cervix any further. The doctor with whom I consulted agreed that a Cesarean section was needed. I felt bad but knew that in this case the Cesarean was necessary. I held Marlene's hand under the blue paper operating room drapes as her healthy baby girl was delivered surgically just before 1 a.m. and left for home as she was being wheeled into the recovery room.

Checking on my patient the next morning I was surprised to find her alone in a private room since she was a clinic patient. Tears formed glistening tracks on her brown cheeks as she lay on her side, arms clasped against her abdomen, writhing in pain. The call bell for the nurse dangled uselessly from the side rail of her bed.

"What?" I signed, holding hands palm up, hunching my shoulders and querying with raised eyebrows.

"Pain," Marlene signed, the tips of her index fingers meeting and separating.

From an IV bag fluid dripped into a vein in her left forearm, but there was no pain medication mixed in. After Cesarean surgery mothers routinely received an intravenous line holding a solution of a powerful narcotic. It was attached to a pump that delivered the medicine in a slow drip; the patient could press a button to get extra painkiller if needed. This patient-controlled analgesia also has the anxiety-relieving effect of putting the patient in charge of her own pain relief, not having to wait for a nurse to give her the medication. Patients often use less analgesic drugs when they can give themselves small, frequent doses.

Every Cesarean post-op patient in this hospital received a patient-controlled analgesia pump – except for the deaf mother who needed it most since verbal communication was so difficult. Marlene's speech, like that of many people who have been deaf since early childhood, was a hard to understand monotone.

My right hand formed a fist that circled my heart, the sign for "Sorry." Then I rushed to the nurses' station.

"The patient in Room 412 needs pain meds right away. Who is her nurse?" I asked as I pulled Marlene's chart from the rack to check the doctor's notes. There was an order for an injection of the narcotic Demerol every 4 hours as needed, but none had been given since the surgery the previous night. Had anyone explained to Marlene how to ring the bell to request pain medication? And how would she have been able to hear the questions asked over the intercom in response to her summons?

After the nurse, Ms. Greene, gave the injection I asked her why Marlene had not been put on a pump for pain meds.

"The anesthesiologist said it would not be appropriate to put her on the patient-controlled pump because he couldn't communicate with her about how to use it properly."

"Marlene is deaf but she can read and write perfectly well," I said, suppressing an angry rant. "Could you please put a pad and pen next to her bed, then there won't be any problem communicating."

"Good idea," she said. "And we've got lots of printed handouts I can give her, baby care, breastfeeding, everything."

Then I explained to Ms. Hopkins, the ward clerk, that my patient was deaf. "If she buzzes the call bell somebody needs to go to her room to see what she needs. She can't hear what you say over the intercom."

"Nobody told me that," Ms. Hopkins said, shaking her head. "Poor mother, going all night without even an aspirin after she's been cut open."

Returning to Room 412 I saw the Demerol was already giving Marlene blessed relief. She was fast asleep.

The anesthesiologist who usually worked on Labor and Delivery was skilled and intelligent. He politely introduced himself to both private and clinic patients.

"I'm Dr. Braun," he would say, flexing his thin arm and pointing to the bicep, "like brawn." With a smile he promised, "We're going to take all your pain away… But you have to do exactly what I tell you," was the stern postscript as he warned the mother not to move a muscle during the procedure. To me his bedside manner seemed condescending but to a woman in pain he was the angel of mercy. His epidurals always worked. In an emergency he could put the patient under general anesthesia in a flash, intubating her with a graceful motion of his wrist while methodically reporting on her condition to the surgeons waiting to cut her baby out of the womb.

I was disappointed that such a smart doctor had been unable to find a way to think outside of his usual routine to provide post-op pain relief to my deaf patient. He had managed to communicate with Marlene when he gave the anesthesia before her surgery. Why not afterward?

And I felt that I shared the blame for not anticipating this problem when the Cesarean had been done. I had failed to look at – or in this case listen to – the situation from the patient's perspective.

Jahaira

Jahaira was completely at home in her pregnant but still tomboyish body. During labor she sounded like a Wimbledon tennis player, not shy about making noise that reflected the hard work she was doing. Between contractions she was totally relaxed, dozing while the endorphins flowed. When it came time to push her baby out she sat up, grabbed her thighs behind bent knees, breathed like a runner before a sprint and grunted with each effort. When her son was born, covered with blood and vernix, the cream-cheese like coating that protects the fetus, she grabbed him with both hands, unafraid of slime. He screamed to fill his lungs with oxygen and she shouted her triumph. Behind the surgical mask I smiled. She probably was one of the patients who wanted to see her placenta when I offered that option, and didn't reply with a disgusted "Yuck."

I went to check on her the next day: she was sitting cross-legged on the bed, her son nursing blissfully at the small left breast half hidden under a sports team t-shirt.

"He loves my titty," Jahaira boasted. She was right about that. The baby's cheeks worked like miniature bellows sucking at her nipple. Soon he was satisfied and fell asleep, a few drops of milk drooling from the corner of his half-open mouth. His milk-filled belly peeked out between his undershirt and diaper. A yellow plastic clamp was still attached to the inch-long stump of umbilical cord, stained deep blue from the antiseptic used to prevent infection around the navel. Jahaira flung him over her shoulder, where he slumped, sated and exhausted, while his mother thumped his back to burp him. His head lolled against her shoulder and I noticed his straight black hair had been combed up into a small Mohawk. After a loud burp broke from his lips, Jahaira put the baby in his bassinet then climbed into bed for my check-up. Her uterus was firmly contracted and she was barely bleeding. A small laceration in her perineum that I had closed with two stitches was clean and intact. Breastfeeding was obviously going well and she handled the baby with confidence. She was fine.

"It's better to sit with your legs together," I told her, "for the stitches to heal."

"Sure," she said.

As I write about her so many years later, it suddenly occurs to me: I wonder if Jahaira was gay. In spite of having lesbian friends and co-workers I often failed to pick up on a woman's sexual orientation. Unless there was some fairly obvious sign to the contrary I generally assumed that a woman having a baby was heterosexual. I remember once haranguing a patient about the need for contraception.

"I'm not going to get pregnant," she said.

"How can you be sure," I asked, "if you don't use birth control?"

"Don't worry, I won't," she insisted.

Raised eyebrows expressed my skepticism.

"I'm gay," she finally blurted out in exasperation, yanking me out of my heterosexist mindset.

"That's an effective method," I said.

Did she smile or was she still peeved by my clueless lecturing? I don't remember.

Tiffany

Tiffany had started prenatal care in Brooklyn but in her sixth month switched to Roosevelt Hospital when she moved in with a relative living nearby. She brought her medical record, which contained information about her check-ups with the previous doctor and all the blood test reports.

Tiffany was 22 and having her first baby. Most of the data in her chart documented an uncomplicated pregnancy. She did not have high blood pressure or diabetes, was of average weight, did not smoke, drink or use drugs. An ultrasound confirmed her early June due date and showed normal fetal anatomy. But there was one worrisome item: a positive test for syphilis. [See Notes to the Reader.] Since she was allergic to penicillin, the best anti-syphilis drug, she had been treated with erythromycin, a less effective antibiotic.

Years earlier at Lincoln a patient I delivered had suffered a tragic and preventable stillbirth caused by syphilis. That experience weighed on my mind as I cared for Tiffany, worrying that the treatment with erythromycin was not effective enough to cure her and prevent her baby from becoming infected.

In 1991, before the internet made researching diseases simple, I relied on my "Bible" – a dog-eared copy of a government pamphlet published every few years called the *Centers for Disease Control Sexually Transmitted Diseases Treatment Guidelines*. The section on syphilis in pregnancy warned that erythromycin was not sufficient for treating the fetus of a penicillin-allergic mother. It recommended allergy testing to be sure the woman really was allergic to penicillin. If she was, the next step was allergy desensitization so she could be treated with the most effective drug.

Many people believe they have an allergy when they have experienced an unpleasant side effect such as nausea and vomiting after taking a pill or redness at the site of an injection. A true allergy is much more serious and involves welts or hives and itching, wheezing, and, in the worst cases, swelling that can lead to a blocked airway and death. Tucked between the pages of my *Treatment Guidelines* were forms for reporting STDs to the Health Department for purposes of contacting the patient's sex partners for treatment and for keeping statistics. It was a time-consuming bit of paperwork, but an important public health measure.

When I explained my concern to Tiffany, she agreed to go to the hospital's allergy clinic for testing, which involved injecting a tiny amount of penicillin under her skin to see if that provoked an allergic reaction or not. The testing has to be done in a place which can provide emergency care in case the patient has a severe reaction. I called the allergy clinic and convinced them to squeeze my patient in that week.

After the appointment, a nurse from the allergy clinic called me on Labor and Delivery to let me know the results were negative – Tiffany was not allergic to penicillin.

"Great," I said. "Please tell the patient to wait for me. I'll be there in five minutes to give her the injection." The labor room was not busy; I would not be missed. I grabbed a vial of the medication, a syringe and needle, alcohol swabs and latex gloves, and hurried to the allergy clinic. The nurse pointed me to an examining room down the hall where Tiffany sat swiveling in an office chair on wheels.

"Are you going to give me the shot now?" she asked.

"The sooner we treat the syphilis the better it is for you and the baby," I said, taking the equipment out of my lab coat pocket and placing it on a small table to draw up the medication. The type of penicillin given for syphilis is a thick white paste, like Elmer's glue, that must be injected with a long, large-bore needle. To the patient it looks quite alarming, so I kept my body between Tiffany and the needle. No point in getting her all nervous while she watched me draw the medicine from the vial into the syringe. I prided myself on being able to give this kind of injection with minimum pain, high on the hip where there is plenty of muscle to absorb the drug and fewer nerves.

"Please pull down your pants and lean over that examining table," I said.

"What?" said Tiffany, "you want to give the shot in my butt?"

"Yes," I said over my shoulder, still trying to keep the syringe out of sight. "It's not so bad. All my patients say I have soft hands." That was true.

"Not in my butt." She was adamant. "Give it in my arm." She rolled up her sleeve to expose this preferred site and stayed planted in the swivel chair.

"There's not enough meat on your arm," I said. "The needle will go in one side and out the other."

"I'm sorry," Tiffany said. "I know you want to help me, but I just can't stand getting a shot in my butt."

I turned to face her, giving up all efforts to conceal the needle, and sat down in a chair opposite her. I looked at her; she looked at me. Then our eyes slid off in different directions. I had spent a lot of time and effort getting the allergy testing arranged and felt angry that Tiffany was suddenly so cowardly about getting an injection. Then I took a deep breath. No point arguing. People have deeply held feelings and fears about where they are touched. Rational explanations cannot overcome those emotions. We sat there for what seemed like a very long minute. She swiveled her chair in semicircles.

Then I had an inspiration. "How about here on your leg?" I pointed to the fleshy quadriceps muscle on the front of my own thigh, remembering this is the place where we give injections to newborn babies.

"No problem," said Tiffany. She pulled her elastic-waist maternity pants down below her knees. I cleansed the skin on her thigh with an alcohol swab and gave the injection. She watched the needle go in and didn't even wince.

"That wasn't too bad," she said, pulling the pants back up over her big belly. "I just can't stand the idea of a shot in my butt."

"You made that clear," I thought, depositing the syringe and needle in the special red plastic receptacle used for disposing of sharp instruments.

"That needle does look scary," I said. "It takes a brave woman to be a mother." My anger and frustration had evaporated. "You can take some Tylenol if your leg hurts… When you come back to prenatal clinic we'll do a blood test to see if the syphilis is gone."

That test showed Tiffany had been cured. Two months later she gave birth to a healthy son.

CHAPTER 8

HIV clinic, 1992–94 Taking on the monster

On November 7, 1991 Magic Johnson announced to a stunned press conference that he was infected with the AIDS virus.

"We sometimes think only gay people can get it, that it's not going to happen to me. And here I am saying it can happen to anybody." Quitting the LA Lakers, Johnson became a spokesperson about HIV and AIDS, warning young people that "safe sex is the way to go."

Johnson's courageous action more than two decades ago was an important moment in the fight against AIDS – and for me. About to begin working in a clinic for HIV-infected women and their children, I wanted Magic's openness to help shatter the secrecy and shame surrounding the epidemic. I was filled with hope that as a midwife caring for pregnant HIV-positive women and doing research on preventing transmission of the virus to their babies I could help avert the suffering this disease wreaked on millions of people worldwide. I had watched several friends shrivel and die of AIDS. I wanted to be on the front line of the battle against this monster. In the early 1990s the few medications available were paltry weapons, pebbles thrown at tanks. But I was ready to throw those pebbles with all my might until we discovered something more powerful.

Friends asked me about possible danger. That was a concern: blood and amniotic fluid that harbor the virus are always part of birth. But for many years I had been practicing "universal precautions," meaning donning gloves, gown, face mask and eye shields to protect myself. It did not matter what the perceived risk status of a patient might be – a nice married lady or a drug user – I protected myself at each delivery. Some midwives felt that such protective garb was a barrier to their relationship with patients. Did they really believe patients cared – or even noticed – what the person catching their baby wore? To me, respecting my patients, and myself, meant practicing the same precautions with everyone.

In the opening days of 1992 I began working at the Center for Mother and Baby Care (a pseudonym for the clinic to protect patient privacy). For the next thirty months I was plunged into the world of AIDS. A new vocabulary of T-cells and opportunistic infections became part of my everyday language. My fingers learned to detect swollen lymph glands less than half an inch in diameter. I taught patients how to use the female condom and set up electronic pillboxes to remind them when to take their medications. I recruited pregnant women into a research trial known as "076" on preventing mother-to-baby HIV transmission. Along with my co-workers I was thrilled and gratified when, in 1994, our study demonstrated how this could be done – the first big breakthrough in AIDS prevention.

Center for Mother and Baby Care

Rose-pattern white lace curtains filtered the dim light from the big window looking out on an air shaft. The three panels of an old-fashioned folding screen were covered with African fabric in bright shades of yellow, magenta, green and black. A poster of Paris and photos of women and babies decorated the pale green walls; a hanging plant trailed down from a pipe.

A desk lamp lit the small rectangular room with a soft glow; long fluorescent ceiling bulbs with their faint hum were switched on occasionally when bright light was necessary. A bed, a desk, two chairs and a small bookcase completed the furnishings. Three brass hooks on the door held coats and other garments.

Yet the homey touches could not mask the purpose of the space. This was a hospital office and examining room. Women learned terrible things here: terrible, frightening things that changed their lives, things to be kept secret and hidden. In my pretty room pregnant women were told they were infected with HIV, the AIDS virus. They were told the babies they carried might also be infected. That is what we told them. What they heard was perhaps something else.

In 1992 many people believed HIV was a man's disease: gay men, drug-injecting men, hemophiliacs. AZT was the only drug available. No protease inhibitors, no non-nucleoside reverse transcriptase inhibitors, no triple therapy nor 4-in-1 pills existed back then. HIV equaled AIDS equaled death, was what most women thought when we told them they had tested HIV positive on routine prenatal blood work. They assumed their baby was also doomed. When we told a patient that her baby had a 25 percent chance of being infected – but that three out of four infants would be HIV negative – they hung on to that shred of hope.

All the babies of HIV-positive mothers are born with antibodies to the virus passed to them from their mothers during pregnancy. It takes about a year for the babies who are not themselves infected to clear these antibodies and test negative. Some of the infected children start showing symptoms of disease within months after they are born, others appear healthy for years. Today, a test to detect the presence of the virus in the blood can determine soon after birth whether or not an infant is infected, but in the early 1990s there was a long anxious wait before a symptom-free baby could be declared HIV negative with antibody tests.

Some patients had a trusted person with whom they could share the news of their infection, and brought them to appointments where we drew blood, explained the disease and options for treatment and gave them a chance to ask questions and talk.

"This is my mother … sister …best friend," they would say, "You can tell her everything."

Others felt there was nobody to whom they could safely reveal their secret. Terrified of the rejection, abandonment or violence which they were sure their HIV status would bring, they lived in isolation. But we, the clinic staff, already knew. Patients clung to us in the days and weeks after they first learned their diagnosis. They might hate us for the bad news we brought them, but they did not have to hide their secret from us.

Those of us working in the clinic were also targets of the fear and prejudice surrounding AIDS. On Labor and Delivery or the postpartum wards the staff called us "the AIDS ladies." When we went there to care for our mothers, someone would often take us aside to whisper, "She seems like a nice lady. How did she get it?"

"Same way she got pregnant," was our standard answer.

Several of my co-workers did not tell their friends, or even their families, that they worked with HIV patients. The benign name of our clinic, the Center for Mother and Baby Care, contained no frightening words or acronyms, revealed nothing of its true purpose.

Treating infected women and their children in the same place was a great innovation. Mothers overwhelmed by their children's needs often neglected their own health. While the kids were with the pediatric nurse practitioners who provided most of the care, the midwives would wheedle the mothers, "You're here now, why not come into my office for a quick check-up." Patients could get all their health care, social services, psychological counseling, even dental check-ups and acupuncture, and enroll in HIV research studies in one place.

The atmosphere was welcoming: a bubbling coffee pot, snacks, toys, small gifts, parties every Halloween and Christmas. The almost all-female staff had worked here for years and knew every patient, greeted them by name and scooped up the children for hugs and kisses. Most patients looked healthy. Nothing proclaimed "AIDS." This was very different from the general HIV clinic downstairs at-

Laboring:

tended almost entirely by men. The gaunt bodies there frightened our patients. The women could not bear to see their future that way. Bringing their children to such a place was unthinkable.

Our patients ran the gamut of risk factors for infection. Some had injected drugs or smoked crack cocaine and were shocked, but not surprised, by a positive HIV test result. The people they knew from the streets were also sick, dying or dead. Some took the HIV diagnosis as a last call to get their lives together, supported by the many services of the clinic. Others fell more deeply into drugs and would disappear for long periods of time, only showing up when they were desperately sick.

Many women had no history of drug use, and only one, two or at most three sex partners in their lives. The virus came from a boyfriend or husband they had never imagined carried a deadly disease.

"He wasn't gay or bisexual as far as I knew," they might say when we queried them about possible sources of infection. "Needles? No, not that I could tell." Or, "He looked clean, healthy."

Several of the women suffered from mental illness, some treated and others not. A small number had been infected by transfusions before the development of HIV antibody testing, approved by the Federal Drug Administration on March 3, 1985, made the blood supply safe. Some of our patients came from African countries where the virus was as prevalent among females as males.

The drug users and former addicts frightened me. I was not afraid they would hurt me – although I always made sure to keep my purse locked up. It was the terrible lives they led, the many forms of abuse they suffered, and the cunning which enabled them to survive. They were smarter than me in a hundred ways and could see right through my professional exterior into every weakness and indecision in my soul.

"No problem," she would say when I handed a user a cup and requested a urine specimen for drug testing, "soon as I can pee." The cup remained empty.

Diane, the other midwife, was much better than I was with the tough ladies. One of our patients, whose scarred body had seen the inside of prisons, mental institutions and rehab facilities told me, "Nobody knows how to yell at me like Diane." There could be no higher praise. Diane instructed this woman on the proper way to do dozens of things, from using deodorant, to putting her medications in a weekly pill container, to holding her newborn son in a sitting position to burp him.

"She never had a mother to teach her," Diane said.

Diane and I are very different. I am petite, soft spoken and dislike conflict. Tall and energetic, with big hands and a strong voice, my co-worker never seemed afraid to speak her mind. She was always ready to play Santa or Mrs. Claus at the Christmas parties that all the patients attended. At the bar across the street from the hospital her Halloween costume as the Condom Queen aka Ms. Safe Sex, consisting of dozens of multi-colored condoms festooning her clothes, was legendary.

Diane came from England, growing up in the working-class town of West Hartleypool, and never lost her British accent.

"You wench!" was Diane's favorite reproach, perhaps to a patient who had missed two appointments and then called requesting to be seen the same day because she needed more birth control pills.

"Don't get your knickers in a twist," was her advice to someone becoming upset or impatient.

"Why did you become a midwife?" I once asked her.

"When I was 11 years old I had a perforated eardrum so I had to be hospitalized for a week with penicillin injections," she told me. "I was the oldest one in the children's ward, so they had me helping with the little ones and making beds. By the end of the week I knew I was meant to be a nurse."

Graduating from high school, Diane entered basic nursing training at the local general hospital. "I went on to midwifery as an extra certification, in a town called Sunderland." After two weeks of midwifery Diane was hooked. "I said this is what I want to do for the rest of my life." She worked there in the 1960s. Wearing the distinctive raincoat of her profession, Diane carried a big black bag with supplies as she rode the bus to deliver babies at home. That was the normal way for English mothers to give birth then. The hospital was for sick people, not for women bursting with new life. The birth control pill had just been developed but was not yet widely used. Big families were common; there were plenty of babies to catch.

Patients sometimes tried to play Diane and me off against one another. If she didn't like my advice, a patient might go to Diane for a "second opinion," or vice versa. Our often identical answers made patients suspect we had talked to each other before responding. But no consultation was needed; we both practiced the same way.

"Should I really take these antibiotics? Won't they hurt my baby?" a pregnant woman might ask me after getting a prescription from Diane.

"She knows you are pregnant and gave you pills that are safe for your baby." I'd answer. "If you don't take these antibiotics the urine infection could get into your kidneys and even cause premature labor. That would be much worse."

"That's what Diane told me," the patient would say, as if surprised to hear near-identical words from midwives with such different personalities.

Whenever Diane learned that a patient from our clinic had been admitted anywhere in the hospital – to medicine, psych, the AIDS ward – she would go to see her, more as a friend than as a professional. She would bring encouragement and body lotion, give massages, wipe off and organize the bedside tray, tidy sheets and blankets. Even as the patient's life was reduced to the few square feet of half a hospital room, Diane would bustle to make everything neat and proper within that small space.

Diane brought a critically ill woman the Chinese meal she craved. The patient was too weak to lift a fork, so my co-worker fed her. I am sure that any bit of food dribbling out of the sick lady's mouth was quickly wiped away by my friend and no grains of rice were left stuck to the pristine bedside tray.

"She enjoyed every bite," Diane said. It was the woman's last meal; she died the next day.

How did Diane cope with all this? "I bury my emotions til I go home," she would say. "Then I have a gin and tonic and think about things."

My feelings were more on the surface and could not be postponed until after work. I remember the birth of Donna, the first of my HIV prenatal patients whom I delivered. Paged to the labor room early on a Saturday morning I arrived just in time to tell her, "You're ready to push this baby out." It was an easy birth. But as I handed Donna her squalling daughter I was swept by a wave of emotion. It was as if I could feel every doubt and regret the mother was experiencing: Do I dare to love this baby who may die and break my heart? And its flip side: when am I going to die and leave my baby a motherless child?

Jeremiah

Jeremiah was eight or nine years old, but small for his age. The lines that ran from the sides of his nose to the corners of his mouth made him look like a little old man. He always carried a backpack; I think it was decorated with cartoon characters or superheroes. From the backpack's top flap plastic tubing snaked over his left shoulder and crept up toward his nose. Twin prongs clipped the tubing to his nostrils. Even with this boost of oxygen the stringy muscles in his thin neck worked hard and popped out with every breath.

The first time I saw Jeremiah was the day I came to the Center for Mother and Baby Care to interview for a job. His little old man face pierced my heart and was part of the reason I accepted the position.

Jeremiah had been born in the mid 1980s. AIDS was considered a disease of gay men back then. The idea that women – and the babies in their pregnant bodies – could also become infected was not well known, even within medical circles. Some denied that such infection was possible, even though other sexually transmitted diseases like syphilis, gonorrhea or chlamydia were passed between men, women and children in the womb. Jeremiah was a living rebuke to the deniers. Having survived this long – before the development of the many drugs that today make HIV a chronic disease rather than a fatal one – he was something of a miracle child.

He visited the clinic often for blood tests and respiratory treatments to help his breathing. We could hear his little boy voice, negotiating with the pediatric nurse practitioner:

"Not that vein, Lillian. You stuck me there last time."

"Where then?" she would ask, holding his brown stick-figure arms, turning them over, inspecting for a place to insert the tiny butterfly needle into a barely visible vein. Sometimes, like a miniature drug addict looking for a new place to shoot up, he would present an untapped vein in an ankle or on the top of a foot.

"How about here?" he would say. "Will it hurt there?" He never cried or had to be held down.

When he was admitted to the Pediatric Intensive Care Unit for his last days, his nurse practitioner spent many hours at Jeremiah's bedside.

"He's more afraid of being alone than of dying," she said.

I wondered if it bothered him that, with the side rails up, the bed looked like a crib.

Many of us from the clinic went to view Jeremiah's body before he was buried. It was the first time I had attended a wake for a child, but would not be the last. The funeral parlor in Harlem reeked of air freshener. The walls were flimsy sheetrock. Several floral arrangements on metal stands stood alongside the small coffin. Comforting thoughts, words like "safe in the arms of Jesus" or "forever in our hearts" were inscribed on ribbons adorning the wreaths. Was he wearing a suit, his dressed-for-church clothes? Was there a teddy bear in his hands? The details have grown fuzzy over the years. But I will never forget the miniature toy car pinned to the white satin lining of Jeremiah's coffin.

The family members and a few friends spoke in low murmurs, sniffled into tissues. Those of us from the clinic did the same. It was all very subdued. Nobody sobbed aloud or cried out about the injustice of a child's death. Nobody mentioned AIDS.

As we filed out of the funeral parlor into the winter night Diane said, "Who wants to go for a drink? I need a gin and tonic." But it was cold and getting late. Tomorrow was a work day. None of us knew where to go in that neighborhood, long before gentrification brought chic bars to Harlem. We drifted toward our cars or the subway station and scattered.

This would be one of many funerals for children that my co-workers and I attended before treatment to prevent transmission of the virus from mother to baby was discovered.

Stuck

When my beeper went off I jumped as if jolted by a small electric shock. It was the first Sunday of the New Year; John and I were eating supper, probably leftovers from a big holiday meal I'd prepared. Midwives and nurses in the clinic shared being on call for our patients' deliveries. Having no plans to party I had volunteered to carry the pager during New Year's week.

"Shit," I said, recognizing the phone number of the labor room. The nurse who answered my call told me that Ms. Alvarez had been admitted. The patient was scheduled to have a repeat Cesarean section later that week but was now in early labor.

"The doctors are planning to operate in about an hour," she said. "How soon can you get here?"

"An hour is fine," I answered, hanging up to call the car service that the clinic hired to ferry patients and staff between home and hospital.

"Quince minutos," (fifteen minutes) the dispatcher told me through the crackling two-way radio that connected her to the fleet of black cars that serve neighborhoods where yellow cabs are rarely found.

Ms. Alvarez was not a patient of mine in the 076 study and the doctors would perform the Cesarean, so my only responsibility would be to obtain extra tubes of blood from the umbilical cord after the placenta was delivered. I finished the last few bites of the meal, put my ID badge around my neck and bundled up against the freezing January night. The car arrived as promised. Traffic on the streets was sparse. I looked out at the holiday lights twinkling across the city as the car enveloped me in soft merengue music and pine air freshener.

At the hospital I changed into scrubs, put on a waterproof gown, shoe covers, cap and mask, and two pairs of sterile gloves. On a stand in the operating room I set up a small metal rack holding six glass test tubes with rubber stoppers. The task was to fill as many of those tubes as possible for testing the baby's blood and storing for future research. A 50 cubic centimeter syringe with a large bore 18 gauge needle was used for drawing up the blood. That's about the size of the big needle used when donating a pint of blood.

The doctors performed the Cesarean quickly, delivering a baby boy with a good Apgar score but whose HIV status would not be known for more than a year. Then they removed the placenta, put it in a blue plastic bowl and handed it to me. There was a foot-long piece of umbilical cord attached. I maneuvered the needle into the vein, the largest of the three vessels in the cord, and pulled back the plunger of the syringe with my right hand to draw out as much blood as possible. I only managed to fill the syringe about half way, but that was good enough. Then I inserted the needle into the rubber stopper of the first tube. The vacuum in the test tube drained blood from the syringe. As the tube became nearly full, I removed the needle and repeated the procedure with the next tube. The suction power of the vacuum sometimes made it hard to withdraw the needle and I had to hold the fourth tube with my left hand while pulling on the syringe with my right. My gloved hands, slick with blood, somehow slipped: I felt the needle prick the index finger of the left hand steadying the tube.

It felt as if time stood still and the freezing winter chill entered my heart. My first thought was "how could I tell my husband he needed to use a condom to protect himself from me?" Then my mind catapulted into a future where I was suddenly transformed from care provider to wraith-like patient. I visualized myself, pale as the sheets on the bed where I lay dying.

I hastily deposited the almost empty syringe in the "sharps" box for safe disposal and rushed to the big scrub sink just outside the operating room. Peeling off the outer glove from my left hand I held it open under a running faucet. Water immediately streamed through the hole made by the needle. Then I took off the inner glove and repeated the test. The heartbeat pounding in my ears was louder than the water gushing out of the faucet. The second glove filled like a balloon. No water flowed out; this glove was intact. The bloody needle had not pierced it.

But that did not stop me from shaking as I vigorously scrubbed my hands with antiseptic soap for several long minutes.

Ms. Alvarez was wheeled into recovery; the baby was in newborn nursery; the tubes of blood were on their way to the lab. My work for this night was done. It was only 11 p.m. but I treated myself to car service home rather than taking the subway. How different the lights across the city seemed now, glittering with menace. What if I had really been stuck?

The next morning I discussed what had happened with the clinic manager and filed an incident report. Co-workers shared needle stick stories; one nurse was pregnant when she got stuck and spent nerve-wracking months not knowing if she and her baby had been infected. We devised a safer way of collecting cord blood. My HIV tests that day, and again three, six and twelve months later, were negative.

I never told John, or anybody outside of the hospital, about this near-miss until twenty years later, when I wrote this story.

Amina

Tall and erect, Amina walked gracefully into the room. With flawless chocolate skin, elegantly braided hair and perfect ivory teeth she carried herself like a queen, outfitted like a model in a custom-sewn dress of colorful print fabric. But Amina was neither royalty nor a celebrity. She was a teenage country girl from a small West African village. Within a year or two she would learn both English and French, but on the day we met she spoke only the language of her region. Could she read or write in her local tongue? I cannot remember. Perhaps she signed her name with an X.

There were many forms to fill out, so many questions for me to ask and for her to answer. Her husband, more than a decade older, translated. Amina was newlywed, recently arrived in New York and pregnant with her first baby. She had enrolled early for prenatal care, surmounting bureaucratic hurdles, barriers of language and culture, offering the vein in her left arm for blood tests. Such pretty-colored stoppers on the tubes – red, gold, lavender, and green.

The red-top tube exploded her world when it revealed antibodies to HIV, human immunodeficiency virus, the AIDS virus. Birth and death embrace tightly in the moment when a pregnant woman learns that she has conceived a new life but has also contracted a fatal disease.

Did she recoil and cry out "no"? Did she protect herself with incomprehension while turning her eyes questioningly to the man who infected her? I was not there when a nurse and social worker told Amina the results of her blood test. We met a week later for her first complete prenatal check-up. Lack of a common language required filtering our words through her husband as translator. When he stepped outside the room during the physical exam, I pantomimed "take off your clothes," "put on this gown," "open your mouth," "take a deep breath." With smiles, gestures and touch we bonded more quickly than with words.

At a later visit, where we would take an extensive social history, including details about sexual partners and drug use, the clinic contacted an organization that worked with West African immigrants to arrange for a translator. It was not proper for her husband to be present when we asked these questions. During the interview, however, I began to feel anxious about Amina's privacy. Few people from her country lived in New York at that time. I was afraid the couple's HIV status might be leaked by the translator and exposed in the small community that spoke the same language. I don't think this happened – the translators were highly professional – but I worried about the possibility.

According to the criteria in use in 1992 for HIV-positive pregnant woman, she was too healthy to require any medication. [See Notes to the Reader.] Amina and her husband decided not to participate in the research we (along with several other sites) were conducting to see whether AZT could reduce mother-to-child transmission of the virus. The name of the study was AIDS Clinical Trial Group 076. Participants received either the medication or placebo (neither patient nor care providers knew which) in pill form during pregnancy and in intravenous form during labor. The newborn was given the same medication as its mother in a pediatric-dose syrup for the first six weeks of life.

Many patients objected strongly to subjecting themselves and their babies to an experiment using drugs in pregnant women. My efforts at recruiting women into 076 sometimes ran into a wall of fear and mistrust. Some referred to the Tuskegee study, in which African American men suffering from syphilis were never offered a cure so that researchers could continue studying the "natural history" of the untreated disease. However, almost all our patients were willing to give extra tubes of blood, be examined or answer questions for studies that did not involve experimental drugs. They fervently hoped science and research would discover some way out of the nightmare of AIDS.

Amina's pregnancy progressed without problem. The fetus grew nicely, along with the young mother's knowledge of English. When I praised her expanding vocabulary she introduced me to her teacher: "Television." After a few months she was independent enough to come to prenatal visits alone on the subway.

The weekly clinic staff meeting was in progress when the receptionist knocked on the conference room door and handed me a note with a message from Philomena, the midwife in Labor and Delivery: "Amina admitted, 8 centimeters." My patient was almost ready to give birth.

"Stay here or go to the labor room?" I asked myself. Most of my work in this clinic was prenatal and gynecology or family planning care. I had attended only a handful of births in the last year and was starting to feel rusty and nervous about deliveries. Amina was not enrolled in 076 so I was not needed to administer the study drug; she was in good hands with the midwife on duty in the labor room.

But those were excuses, not reasons. No real midwife would sit in a meeting while her patient was in labor. I excused myself, hurried to Labor and Delivery, and changed into scrubs. Coming out of the locker room I saw Amina's husband pacing back and forth in the hallway. Spotting me he gestured urgently toward the room where his wife was about to deliver. In his culture men did not attend the births of their children.

I put on a mask, cap and shoe covers, quickly scrubbed my hands and pushed the delivery room door open with my shoulder. My hands were held at face level, away from my body and any unsterile surface that might contaminate them.

"Hello, Amina," I said, shrugging a waterproof gown onto my arms and pulling on two pairs of sterile gloves. Glasses protected my eyes from splashes of blood or amniotic fluid.

"Ellen," she sighed, glad for a familiar presence. My face was hidden behind protective gear, only my voice and blue eyes were recognizable.

Philomena had been caring for Amina up to now, but graciously ceded her place at the foot of the delivery table to me. With a few powerful pushes the young mother gave birth to a daughter with a dark halo of fluffy hair and a strong cry.

* * *

In the spring of 1994, the 076 study was closed early due to the clear effectiveness of AZT in preventing mother-to-child viral transmission. One in four babies in the placebo group were infected, compared to only one in twelve who received the medication. It would not be ethical to give the placebo once AZT was proven to greatly reduce the chances of infection in the child. All HIV-positive pregnant women were then offered the medication to protect their babies. Many who had declined to be part of an experimental drug trial gladly accepted the medication once it was proven safe and effective.

When the study ended so did funding for my position as a midwife and researcher. Our contract entitled me to 30-days' notice before being laid off. During that time we called in all the study participants to thank them and say goodbye, and shared with them the now "unblinded" information revealing who had received AZT and who got the placebo.

After two and a half years in the clinic I was burnt out, stressed by the sadness of this work. Sadness and the weight of the secrets about their illness that so many of our patients held close. Attending the funeral of a baby I delivered who had supposedly died of asthma I wanted to scream out the truth. Why didn't the funeral directors who prepared the small corpses and the ministers who prayed for the dead children sound the alarm that AIDS is here, infecting women and babies. Why didn't I?

It was a relief to lose my job. Being laid off was an easy way out – far easier than quitting, abandoning co-workers and patients, and having to admit that this work required a kind of strength and stamina that I lacked. I looked forward to taking the summer off. In the fall I would find another job, a normal midwife job. My husband was teaching mathematics at a community college, earning enough to pay the bills until I began bringing home a paycheck again.

Amina's last visit with me was a routine check-up. We needed no translator.

"My daughter fine," she said of her HIV-negative toddler, now 18 months old. Even without treatment Amina's little girl had escaped infection.

I waited until the end of the visit to tell her I was leaving.

"Diane, the other midwife, will take good care of you," I said as we hugged goodbye. Usually I walked patients from my examining room to the reception desk, giving their medical record to the clerk to make follow-up appointments. But this time I handed Amina her chart and closed the door behind her. I needed to be alone to cry.

A knock on the door half a minute later made me grab some tissues and hastily dry my eyes. I opened the door and saw Amina, wiping her cheeks with the palm of one hand. We clasped each other for real this time, my head resting against her slender neck as our tears flowed and mingled.

With the development of powerful new anti-viral drugs in 1996 Amina remained symptom-free for many years. She may still be alive today, two decades after we first met.

Thank you, my beautiful daughter Amina, for sharing your grace and resilience with me.

CHAPTER 9

Back to normal midwife work, 1994–2005

Soon after being laid off by the HIV clinic I was hired by Columbia Presbyterian to fill a vacancy in the staff of midwives caring for normal prenatal and family planning patients. I was assigned to one of the half dozen outpatient clinics scattered throughout the Washington Heights/Inwood neighborhood. Midwives delivered patients at the Allen Pavilion, a 300-bed community hospital at the northern tip of Manhattan, where the Harlem and Hudson Rivers meet. From the windows of several labor rooms you sometimes saw the Columbia University rowing team practicing on the water just beyond the hospital, their oars dipping and lifting in perfectly synchronized motion.

There were some 2,500 babies born here each year, with midwives delivering about half that number. The Allen Pavilion was part of the big Columbia Presbyterian Medical Center whose main campus was located on and around 168th Street and Broadway. Mothers with uncomplicated pregnancies went to the Allen while high-risk patients delivered at Babies' Hospital (now the Morgan Stanley Children's Hospital) at the main campus. This huge complex, just south of the George Washington Bridge, dominates upper Manhattan and grew even more massive after merging with Cornell University's New York Hospital in 1998. The name of the combined institution became New York Presbyterian Hospital.

Ms. Rodriguez

"The doctor said my pelvis was too narrow," Ms. Rodriguez told me as I took her medical history at her first prenatal visit. "So he had to do a C-section."

"Were you in labor when he decided that?" I asked.

"No. It was a few days before my due date; he told me to come into the hospital for surgery the next morning."

"How much did the baby weigh?" was my next question.

"My son was 6 pounds 14 ounces." That is not a big baby.

I was suspicious of the "narrow pelvis" rationale the doctor had given her. And when I did the vaginal exam I could feel she had a roomy pelvis that could easily birth a much bigger child. It made me angry that women were told such lies about their bodies; and even sadder that they believed these untruths. I wondered about the doctor's motivation. Perhaps he considered spending long hours at the side of a laboring woman a waste of valuable time; it was so much more efficient to schedule surgery at 8 a.m. and be back seeing patients in the office before 10. Maybe he had been sued for malpractice and was now practicing defensive medicine by doing more Cesareans. He might even think, "No harm done."

Generations ago, when childhood polio and the vitamin-deficiency disease rickets were common, girls' pelvic bones became deformed from those illnesses, making childbirth difficult and dangerous. A girl who becomes pregnant at a very young age, before having completed her own growth and development, especially if she is malnourished, may also have an abnormally small pelvis. But of the thousands of women and teenagers I examined over the course of several decades I found a truly narrow pelvis in only two. One of them was able to give birth vaginally to a smallish baby of about 5 ½ pounds. The other had such a reduced pelvis that normal delivery would have been impossible: I immediately transferred her to an obstetrician.

There are many reasons why a Cesarean section may be needed to preserve the health or even the life of a mother or baby. But in 21st century United States a narrow pelvis is rarely a valid cause.

I mentioned to Ms. Rodriguez the possibility of having a vaginal birth with this baby. She had not known that option existed. As her pregnancy progressed we discussed it again. We sent away for the record of her Cesarean to check the kind of incision that had been made in her uterus. A horizontal cut into the lower part of the womb makes it safe to go through labor for a subsequent birth. A vertical incision, cutting into the part of the uterine muscle which contracts during childbirth, would rule out a vaginal birth. The scar on her abdomen was a "bikini cut" and the more important uterine incision was the horizontal kind. It would be safe to go through labor.

In her eighth month Ms. Rodriguez was still unsure whether to schedule a repeat Cesarean or wait to go into labor on her own and try for a vaginal birth. Her pregnancy was healthy and without complications.

"Taking care of a baby was hard when I was just healing from surgery," she said of her first delivery. "It will be even harder with an active 4-year-old at home too." She finally decided to try for a normal birth, or a "trial of labor" in medical terms. I did a vaginal exam as her due date approached.

"The baby's head is deep down in your pelvis," I reported, truthfully, to boost her confidence in her body's ability to birth this child. "There's plenty of room for him or her to be born vaginally."

I was not in Labor and Delivery when she was admitted a few days later, but saw her on the postpartum floor the next morning. She was tired after an exhausting night in labor. A rosy-faced baby girl slept swaddled in blankets in the clear plastic bassinet next to her bed.

"I did it, Ellen. I gave birth naturally!"

In my heart I cheered for her, but did not want my enthusiastic response to influence her account of the birth.

"How was it?" I asked.

"Pretty rough at times. I needed stitches too. But the pushing wasn't bad. And once the baby was out the pain was over."

Now I could let my praise fly.

"You did great! How big is she?" The baby's weight was printed on a pink card taped to the bassinet, but I wanted to hear Ms. Rodriguez say it herself.

"Eight pounds one ounce, 21 inches long."

Pretty good work for a pelvis "too narrow" to deliver the older brother who weighed a pound less.

A Night in November

The green numbers on the digital clock blinked 1:50 a.m. as the phone jolted me out of a deep sleep.

"Ma," said my daughter Sara, "my bag of water just broke. The contractions are coming every four, five minutes." Her voice was excited, but without the urgency of a woman close to giving birth. This was Sara's first child and she was home alone while her husband was waiting for a visa to come to this country. During the pregnancy Sara had gone to a well-regarded midwife practice that delivered patients at St. Vincent's Hospital in Greenwich Village. Happy for my daughter, and thrilled at becoming a grandmother, I was glad to give her support and advice, but leave the actual prenatal care and delivery to them. When dealing with pregnant relatives or friends I was concerned that our close relationship might cloud my professional judgment, perhaps causing me unconsciously to deny any problem I did not want to see.

"I'll be right there," I said. I brushed my teeth, put on some sweats, grabbed my purse, threw in a camera and was out the door.

It was a freezing November night. No people on the street, few lights in the windows, as I walked the two short blocks to Sara's house. The only sound was the rustling of fallen leaves brushing against my feet. My key to the side door of her building turned,

Laboring:

but did not open the lock. After a few tries I gave up and walked another block to the main entrance. The key did not open this door either. Using the intercom, which worked through the telephone, I rang her apartment. Busy signal.

"She's calling her midwife," I thought. Half a minute later I tried again. Still busy. On the third try she picked up:

"Hurry, ma." She buzzed me in.

The elevator slowly lumbered to the eighth floor. Getting out I heard a baby crying and thought "Sara never mentioned that one of her neighbors has a baby." The door to her studio apartment yielded to my key. My daughter was standing there in her bathrobe, a wet newborn bawling in her arms. Part of me realized this as soon as I heard the crying infant, but another part was not ready to believe it.

"The baby is out," she said.

"I see. What is it?" I asked.

"I haven't checked yet," she answered. We looked together: a girl. The infant's loud cries reassured me her lungs were working just fine.

"Dalia!" Sara greeted her daughter with the name she had chosen.

"Let's get this baby dry and covered, it's cold in here," I said, my midwife persona taking charge. I turned on a lamp in the dark room, dried the black-haired infant and wrapped her in a blanket. Sara put the baby to her breast to nurse. I delivered the placenta and put it in a plastic bag, still connected by the umbilical cord to the newborn. There was no need to cut the cord and nothing sterile with which to clamp and sever it safely. Although shaken by birthing her baby alone Sara was fine except for needing some stitches. She called her midwife back – having abruptly hung up as the baby was born – and arranged to meet her at the hospital. Then I called my husband.

"John, put the baby seat in the car and come pick us up," I said.

"Why do you need the car seat?" he wanted to know.

"Because we have a baby girl here," I answered.

"Is everyone all right?" John asked.

"Yes, Sara and the baby are both fine."

"Then why do they need to go to the hospital?" Spoken like a man who has lived with a midwife and listened to my stories about how normal births don't require all the paraphernalia, or all the germs, a hospital can provide.

"Sara needs some stitches. Her midwife is on her way to St. Vincent's."

Mother, baby and grandmother bundled up and John drove us to the hospital. Sara was put in a private room: a practice based on labeling deliveries outside the hospital as "dirty" and isolating the offenders from the "clean" patients.

When we talked about it afterward, Sara told me she had been really scared, but hearing my voice on the telephone had calmed her down so much that she did not convey the urgency she felt. Usually I can tell from a woman's voice how advanced her labor is, but I failed to hear that with Sara. Then she says of her often tardy daughter, "That was the first and last time Dalia got some-place too early." We laugh together. If Dalia is listening she rolls her eyes. And John still teases me, "You were so busy brushing your teeth you missed the birth."

I prefer to blame the badly copied key to Sara's building for my failure to be with my daughter when she really needed me. As a mother and a midwife I'd missed a major event in my child's life.

In prenatal clinic mothers expecting their first baby often asked, "How will I know when I'm in labor?"

"Don't worry," I replied, "You'll know." None of my patients had ever given birth to a first child at home. The more common scenario was coming to the hospital too soon.

"Wait until the contractions get your complete attention. If you can walk or talk during a contraction you're not ready." It's good advice, but even the best advice is not applicable to every situation.

My granddaughter is now a beautiful young woman getting ready to go to college, but I remember every detail of the November night she was born.

Sara's second child was born at the Allen Pavilion six years later. Wanting to avoid a replay of her first birth experience she went to the hospital a bit too early. Her labor proceeded in its own leisurely way as she alternated between walking the hallways and resting in bed. Sara's midwife did not intervene to speed things up. My daughter birthed a healthy baby boy about twelve hours after being admitted, with her midwife, husband and me at her side the whole time.

Becoming a grandmother surprised me with the intensity of the love I felt for my grandchildren. It comes at a time of life when you don't expect to feel so deeply again. But unlike youthful or even middle-aged passion, loving your grandchildren will not break hearts, scandalize the neighborhood or ruin your reputation. It is all good.

Damaris

Yvonne was glad to see me at 7:30 a.m. as I arrived to relieve her after her 12 1/2-hour overnight shift in Labor and Delivery at the Allen Pavilion.

We sipped the coffee I brought as Yvonne related the events of the night and prepared me to take over. She was weary and her sour breath revealed she had not gotten a moment's break to freshen up, let alone time to put her feet up or her head down. The skin on her hands was dry and rough, an occupational hazard in a profession where washing our hands 40 or more times a day with harsh hospital soap was part of the job.

In the mid-nineteenth century, before it was known that microorganisms cause disease, Austrian doctor Ignaz Semmelweis noticed that patients in the Vienna General Hospital delivered by midwives – who were scrupulously clean – rarely succumbed to deadly fevers after giving birth. He instituted handwashing in a chlorinated solution for doctors, who often went directly from autopsies to deliveries. The result was a sharp decrease in maternal deaths from childbed fever. But accusing doctors of causing death and disease made Semmelweis a pariah. He died in an insane asylum years before the germ theory of disease found acceptance in the scientific community.

Before massaging lotion into her chapped hands, my co-worker squeezed a blob of the cream into my palm. Yvonne dispensed advice and encouragement in both English and Spanish. Unfailingly supportive and upbeat, her skills and teamwork earned everyone's respect. A few months earlier, in the face of the most devastating event possible in Labor and Delivery – a maternal death – Yvonne mined a nugget of hope from the tragedy: that the mother who suffered a postpartum hemorrhage and refused blood transfusion for religious reasons had died true to her faith. The rest of the grieving staff was too angry at the patient for what she did to her orphaned children, and to us, to find comfort anywhere.

I was relieved not to have been in Labor and Delivery that terrible day, but still mourned the death along with every other person in the maternity service.

During the night Yvonne had evaluated six patients who came to the hospital to be triaged for possible admission. Three patients were not in active labor and had no complications, so Yvonne sent them home. Families were often nervous and sometimes resistant to leaving. But admitting a patient too soon might condemn her to a cascade of interventions. Once in the hospital the pressure is on to "get her delivered." Cesarean section for "failure to progress" may result when the real failure was the inability to patiently await the onset of true labor. It is a situation midwives try to avert by giving mothers the knowledge and confidence to stay home in early labor unless some complication makes hospitalization absolutely necessary.

Yvonne had admitted three women and delivered two of their babies in the pre-dawn hours. The third patient was now fully dilated and ready to start pushing her baby out. It was a first baby and the labor was accompanied by elevated blood pressure. The medication given for that had slowed down labor, so Pitocin was started to stimulate stronger and more frequent – as well as more painful – contractions. Epidural anesthesia relieved her pain, but eliminated the urge to push. It was a familiar scenario, and the kind of birth I dreaded. Mothers on this combination of drugs often bleed profusely after the delivery. Mentally I reviewed the emergency measures for postpartum hemorrhage.

Yvonne and I entered the room where the puffy-faced young woman lay in a tangle of IV tubes and wires running from belts around her abdomen to the fetal monitor. One arm was encased in an automatic blood pressure cuff that measured her pressure every few minutes, hissing as the cuff inflated and deflated. Various machines sounded a chorus of beeps. From a catheter in the patient's bladder, clear yellow urine ran into a bag hanging from the bed frame where it could be measured and tested for protein. Her sister stood close by, wiping the laboring woman's face with a wet washcloth. Julia, the nurse just coming on duty, was checking that the various intravenous solutions and medications were being dispensed at the correct rates. There was a round of good morning greetings.

"Damaris," said Yvonne touching the patient on her shoulder, "My shift is over. This is Ellen. She will take care of you now."

"Can't you stay?" said Damaris.

"I've been working all night and I'm exhausted," Yvonne said. "Ellen brings you fresh energy. That's what you need now... Have a beautiful baby." They hugged goodbye.

* * *

"Good morning, Damaris," I said. "It's been a long night but you'll be holding your baby in your arms soon." To Yvonne, who faced a long drive in morning rush hour traffic, "Get home safe."

The monitor indicated that Damaris was having a contraction but she was drowsy and showed no sign of pain, no urge to push. According to Yvonne's examination at 7:24 a.m., the patient's cervix was fully dilated but the baby's head was still high in the pelvis. She estimated the baby weighed about 8 pounds. Rest would be more effective than starting to push too soon and exhausting the mother's strength. The baby's heartbeat was strong; the mother's vital signs were stable. There was no rush. We waited. I massaged Damaris' feet, the sister offered medicine cups filled with ice chips to moisten her dry lips.

About half an hour later Damaris began to feel the urge to push. With the head of the bed raised she pushed in a half-sitting posture for a dozen contractions. The sister, the nurse and I murmured words of encouragement. Nobody shouted "push, push." The only other sounds were the beeps and hisses of the machines, the steady, reassuring beat of the baby's heart amplified by the fetal monitor and the patient's grunts as she pushed.

At my suggestion she then tried lying on her left side, curled around her belly, as I supported her right leg, heavy and numb from the epidural anesthesia. This position helped the baby's head maneuver through the pelvis. With each push we could see a bit of the baby's black hair, but between contractions the head receded.

"I can't do it anymore," Damaris said. "How much longer?"

"You can do it," I said. "We can see the top of the baby's head. Take a break and rest with the next contraction if you want."

"No," she said. "Here comes another one." She put all her strength into that push. More of the baby's head was visible, and stayed that way after the contraction ebbed.

"Good work, mommy. Do you want to feel your baby's head?" I said.

"How?" Damaris asked.

I took her right hand and placed it between her legs on the top of the baby's head. "Like this."

"Is that really his head?" she asked.

"It is," her sister confirmed.

"Yes," I said. "We're getting set up for the delivery right now."

It took another half hour until her baby was born, the nurse, the sister and I all breathing and pushing along with Damaris. It was almost 10 a.m. when I injected local anesthesia and told Damaris I needed to cut an episiotomy to facilitate the birth. Changes in the baby's heartbeat made me decide not to let the pushing phase go on much longer.

"It's a boy," I announced when the chubby newborn was fully delivered. His body felt heavy, close to 9 pounds, as I lifted him onto his mother's belly. He cried right away while Julia dried him with a warm towel.

"My baby, my baby," said Damaris, enfolding her wet, squirming son in her arms.

"What's wrong with the baby's head?" gasped the sister, noticing its elongated, cone-like shape.

"That's normal," I said. "It's called molding. The bones of a baby's head are soft, so they can mold to the shape of the mother's vagina as it squeezes through. Don't worry, tomorrow it will be nice and round."

Several minutes later the placenta delivered, fat and healthy like the baby, along with a gush of blood. I immediately started to massage the mother's abdomen. The nurse injected Pitocin into one of Damaris' intravenous bags and opened the valve to let it flow quickly into the vein. [See Notes to the Reader.]

If the uterus contracts strongly and feels firm to the examiner's hand on the abdomen the patient will not lose too much blood. But Damaris' uterus still felt boggy and she was bleeding heavily from the vagina. The various medications, the long labor and big baby combined produced more bleeding than normal. In the blue basin under the mother's hips a pool of dark red blood almost an inch deep was accumulating. My gut clenched.

"Postpartum hemorrhage. I have to do bimanual compression," I told the nurse, alerting her to the problem and the emergency measure I needed to employ. "Get the doctor," I added, calling for backup in case surgery was needed to stop the bleeding. "And have the blood bank type and cross-match the patient for two units of blood."

"Damaris, this is going to hurt. You are bleeding too much and I have to massage your womb from inside." Putting a sterile glove on my right hand, I curled my fingers into a fist and inserted it into the patient's vagina as gently as possible. Luckily the epidural and local anesthesia blocked most of the pain of this procedure.

With my left hand on her abdomen and the right in her vagina, I massaged and compressed the uterus between them, until I felt it become firm. As I withdrew my right hand I could see that the bleeding had slowed to a trickle.

"Everything under control?" asked the obstetrician responding to the call for help.

"I had to do bimanual compression to stop the bleeding. The uterus is firm now," I told the doctor, "but I need to check the placenta and also see if there are any lacerations."

Watching out for more bleeding with one eye, I carefully examined the placenta. It was intact and complete, all its lobes, like big lumpy pieces of liver, were there, with nothing left inside the mother to cause further hemorrhage or infection. But as I inspected her perineum and vagina I saw that, in addition to the episiotomy I had cut, Damaris had a tear that extended into the muscle of her rectal sphincter. In midwifery training I had learned how to suture this type of tear, called a third degree laceration, but had little practice doing so. A poorly repaired rectal laceration can lead to incontinence, so I asked the obstetrician, who had much more surgical experience, to suture the sphincter. She identified the ends of the torn muscle with clamps and repaired it with a few deft stitches.

Then I finished sewing up the episiotomy. I had given Damaris plenty of local anesthesia and the epidural had not yet worn off. The new mother's gentle snores assured me that my stitching caused no pain as she slept after an exhausting birth.

My back ached when I finally completed the repair, bathed Damaris and put an icepack on her perineum to prevent swelling. As Julia and I made up the bed with clean linens, we saw how much blood saturated the pad and sheets that had been underneath the patient. My blue paper shoe covers left bloody footprints around the bed. I estimated the blood loss at 1,000 cubic centimeters – over a quart – more than twice the normal amount. The mother was stable now, but the heavy bleeding was upsetting.

"Postpartum hemorrhage," I wrote in the chart and documented the bimanual compression used to stanch the bleeding. Routine lab tests done the morning after delivery revealed moderate anemia, but Damaris had no symptoms of weakness or dizziness. The midwife caring for postpartum mothers discharged her home the next day, with advice to eat plenty of rice and iron-rich beans and keep taking her prenatal vitamin pills.

Damaris' delivery replayed many times in my mind, and probably in my unremembered dreams, over the next weeks. It was like watching a movie in slow motion, frame by frame, looking for the one still that might reveal the face of a wrongdoer. What could I have done better? During that time my mind might wander back to the birth as my husband and I chatted. My hands, unconsciously mimicking the motions for delivering a placenta or performing bimanual compression, betrayed my preoccupation.

"Where are you, Ellen?" John would ask. I tried to repeat the last few words of our conversation, hoping to demonstrate that I was paying attention, still there. I tried never to talk about cases with bad outcomes at home, only discussing them with my colleagues. What I shared with family and friends – the "civilians" – were stories with happy endings or descriptions of my frustration with hospital bureaucracy or conflicts with doctors over how to manage a patient.

Many mental re-runs of Damaris' baby's birth revealed no culprit and I finally absolved myself, even as I wondered how the mother was recovering.

About six weeks later I saw Damaris in the hallway of the prenatal clinic. She had just finished a postpartum checkup with the midwife who had cared for her during pregnancy. The puffiness in her face was gone, replaced by the glow of new motherhood.

The rosy undertones of her café au lait skin told me her body had replaced the lost red blood cells and she was no longer anemic. Looking sexy in tight jeans and a flowered top, only a hint of belly showed under her blouse. We hugged and she pulled a photo of her chubby-cheeked son from her purse for me to admire. He had weighed 8 pounds 13 ounces at birth and was more than 11 pounds at his pediatric check-up the previous week.

"We named him Christian," she said.

"Are you getting enough sleep?" I asked. That was usually my first question for new mothers, remembering feeling close to hallucinating from sleep deprivation in the early months after my own children were born.

"Well, he wakes up once or twice during the night to nurse but falls asleep again pretty fast. He's a good baby."

"How was your check-up today?" I asked.

"My midwife says everything is fine," she replied. "She gave me the shot. I don't need another baby anytime soon." 'The shot' is shorthand for Depo Provera, a very effective form of hormonal contraception given by injection every three months.

"Any problem with the stitches?" was my next question and the thing that concerned me most, now that I knew the anemia was resolved.

Damaris looked puzzled. "Stitches? Did I have stitches?" she asked.

"Some," I said, nonchalantly, glad for her amnesia.

Thank you, Damaris, for being young and healthy and recovering completely from a difficult birth.

Marta

Marta missed her six-week postpartum appointment. Between her baby's check-ups and going back to community college to finish her associate degree it was just one thing too many. Besides, she felt great; no need for a check-up. Before leaving the hospital, a nurse gave her an injection, saying, "Don't get pregnant for three months." The new mother assumed she'd received the long-acting contraceptive shot.

Her little boy was about four months old when Marta came to see me, wanting birth control and a bit concerned that, although she'd only nursed for a month, she still hadn't gotten her period.

Marta had been my patient during an uncomplicated pregnancy. Blood tests done at her first visit showed that she had no antibodies to rubella, also called German measles, meaning she had never been infected with or immunized against that childhood disease. I had noted in big letters on her chart that she needed rubella vaccine after delivery. [See Notes to the Reader.]

When Marta described the injection she'd received before her discharge from the Allen Pavilion, I was confused. Had she been given Depo Provera, the injectible contraceptive, as she believed, or rubella vaccine, as I had ordered? Or both?

"It was just one shot," she was sure.

The postpartum nurses kept a vaccination log, recording the date, patient name and the lot number of every immunization given. We needed to be certain if Marta got the vaccine, and was not protected against pregnancy, or if she got the contraceptive shot and still needed rubella vaccine. While dialing the hospital to track down this information I gave Marta a urine cup and a requisition slip for a pregnancy test.

"Give us some urine and take it to the lab," I said. "Then I'll examine you."

The clerk on postpartum answered the phone and promised to have one of the nurses check the vaccination log book and call me back.

When Marta returned and I did a pelvic exam I could feel her uterus, the size of a tennis ball, ten weeks pregnant.

During the exam there was a knock on the door of my examining room; "I have your patient's test results," said Lorena, the medical assistant.

While Marta was putting her clothes on, the postpartum nurse called to confirm that the patient had received the measles, mumps and rubella vaccine. Then I went to the lab where Lorena showed me what I knew would be a positive pregnancy test result.

I wanted to scream, curse and kick something. Before telling my patient she was pregnant I needed to take some deep breaths to cool my anger and frustration. This was not the first time such a serious breakdown in communication had occurred and a patient became pregnant because she thought the immunization she received was a form of birth control. At more than one departmental meeting with doctors, nurses and administrators, midwives had requested that patients be given a clearly written description of the vaccine they received in order to avoid confusion. Our suggestion for a simple solution was either ignored or caught in the eternal limbo of bureaucratic procedures for approving any patient education material.

Leaving the hospital with her newborn, a mother is often anxious, not ready to receive and process more than two pieces of information. Yet she may be overwhelmed with multiple instructions about caring for her baby and herself, follow-up appointments, prescriptions, birth certificate forms, and so forth. The unnecessary admonition "don't get pregnant for three months" was often given along with the rubella vaccination, although there is no evidence that conceiving sooner will cause birth defects. How easy it is for a new mother to interpret that sentence to mean "you won't get pregnant for three months with this injection."

Marta was dressed and waiting for me.

"I'm sorry to tell you there was a misunderstanding about the injection you received. It was not the contraceptive shot, it was a rubella vaccination. You are pregnant, about ten weeks by the size of your uterus."

She looked at me wide-eyed. "How can that be? My son is only four months old... It's too soon."

I nodded, waiting a moment before asking, "What do you want to do?"

"I don't believe in abortion, Ellen," she said, "but I cannot have another baby now."

How many times I had heard that sentence. Almost every patient whose unintended pregnancy threatened to derail her education, work or ability to care for other children used the same words. I'd heard it in English and in Spanish.

"Yes, it is too soon" I agreed. Giving her the name and address of a respected abortion provider I added, "They take your insurance. Make an appointment right away – you are still in the first trimester when it is a simple procedure. But after another two weeks it will become much more complicated."

When I was a nurse at Bellevue patients were admitted to the gynecology unit one day a week for second trimester abortions, called TIP for Therapeutic Interruption of Pregnancy. First, a doctor inserted small dilating sticks called laminaria into the cervix, where they remained overnight to soften and open the mouth of the womb. The next morning labor was induced, often a long and painful process that might take a day or more before the fetus was expelled. At that point the patient was taken to Labor and Delivery.

The staff there, who had to wrap and label the fetuses, hated TIP day. It was a favorite time to call in sick. How easy to feel judgmental and upset – not so much at the young girls who did not even realize they were pregnant until the baby started to kick or someone noticed their growing belly – but at the grown women who delayed and delayed. Each one had her own reasons. As a fervent supporter of a woman's right to abortion I was never punitive in my care after their exhausting and messy ordeal. Sometimes a co-worker could not hide her distress.

"The patient in Room 2 asked what sex it was," said Ms. Martin, a Licensed Practical Nurse. "I told her if she waited another few months and had the baby she would know… Why did she wait so long?"

In the 21st century much of pregnancy care is focused on using sonograms to scan fetal anatomy, amniocentesis and genetic testing to detect Down's syndrome and other abnormalities. These procedures are not just abstract peeks at the baby in the womb. To the provider who orders them or the woman who undergoes these procedures every sonogram or amniocentesis means confronting the possibility of deciding to terminate a pregnancy based on the information the test reveals. What is to be done if a sonogram shows that a large part of the fetal brain is missing or the chambers of the heart are abnormally developed, beyond the ability of any surgeon to repair? What if the fetus is hideously deformed, like the stillborn baby I saw at Bellevue more than thirty years ago and can never forget, with one huge eye in the middle of his forehead? I wrapped him in a blanket, covering his face, and showed the mother one perfectly formed little hand. I could not think what else to do, and everyone else had fled from the room.

The need for abortion is built into the high-tech way modern prenatal care searches for fetal abnormalities. Abortion is also a vital component of women's reproductive rights and the ability to control one's body. I have the greatest respect for the doctors who provide abortions, sometimes at great personal risk, and for the pro-choice advocates and activists fighting to keep abortion legal, safe and accessible.

Morning coffee

To get to my job at the northern tip of Manhattan by 7:30 a.m. required waking up in the dark two hours earlier. I was compulsive about getting to work on time to relieve the midwife who had done the overnight shift, knowing how eagerly I awaited that relief when working nights. Taking public transportation meant needing to allow extra time for the longer interval between subway trains at that early hour, and the possibility of delays.

My husband loyally woke up with me, making cappuccino and breakfast as he listened to re-runs of old Jean Shepherd programs on the radio while I showered and dressed. After I left the apartment at 6:15 a.m. he would go back to sleep or to the gym or check email before leaving for work. His job was three miles from home – in good weather he walked there – and began at a more civilized 9 a.m.

Tuesday was the only day I had the same assignment every week, starting with seeing postpartum mothers at the Allen Pavilion, then taking the hospital shuttle van to the Washington Heights clinic where my patients came for prenatal and family planning care. The other days or nights, including weekends and holidays, I would work in the labor room, or see outpatients for another midwife who was taking vacation or sick leave. Midwives rarely called in sick, often forgoing the paid sick day each month provided for in our union contract.

While covering for the oldest member of our service one time, every co-worker greeted me, eyes widened in amazement, with the identical words: "Doris Barker called in sick? She must be *really* sick!" Her patients were equally surprised and disappointed. "Where's *my* midwife," they pouted. Doris worked into her seventies. She was not just old, she was old fashioned. She spoke only minimal Spanish in an area where that was the primary language. But her patients looked beyond her plain vanilla exterior to the caring and love she extended to them. Their rolling eyes (I could feel them behind my back) and arms crossed over chests – all the body language of their collective rejection of me as a substitute – were a tribute to their *real* midwife, the beloved Ms. Barker.

The driver of the shuttle that ferried us between the Allen Pavilion, community clinics and the main campus on 168th Street on Tuesday morning had a smooth, deep voice and drove skillfully through streets that were an obstacle course of double-parked cars and trucks. He kept the vehicle immaculate and set the van's radio to his favorite music and news. Passengers knew better than to request another station or change in volume. As we rode down Broadway one Tuesday morning just before 9 a.m. the radio reported that a small commuter plane had accidentally flown into one of the Twin Towers.

"The World Trade Center," I cried, "my husband works there!" Then, checking my watch, I added, relieved, "But he's always late to work. He would never be there this early."

* * *

Like all hospitals, Presbyterian had an emergency plan to be implemented in the event of an external disaster that might bring mass casualties to its doors. The plan called for managers to phone the security division for instructions. But on Tuesday, September 11, 2001 many phones were out of service and security did not know what instructions to give. It was almost noon when the hospital administration decided to close the outpatient clinics. Few patients had shown up for appointments anyhow. The workers could go home.

Having managed to contact my husband and children and knowing they were safe I decided to walk back to the Allen Pavilion, a mile away. This was not part of the non-functioning disaster plan, but I wanted to be at the hospital in case staff members on the next shift were unable to get to work. Would public transportation be running? Would highways be shut down? Many co-workers drove across the George Washington Bridge from New Jersey – would traffic be allowed on the bridge? Nobody knew.

Carmela, a night shift nurse who lived in New Jersey arrived just after 7 that evening. Co-workers gathered around to hear her describe how she got to work.

"I put on my white uniform with the hospital ID around my neck and headed for the GWB," she told us. "I had no idea if it would be open or not… As I got closer to the bridge, the police saw my uniform and waved me on. Then I was driving across the river and suddenly it hit me: my car was the only vehicle on the George Washington Bridge."

By 8 p.m. Labor and Delivery was adequately staffed and I could leave. The lavender pants suit I put on that morning was stuffed into a plastic bag. Later for the civilian clothes. Scrubs, a white lab coat and my hospital badge would give me a pass on the streets.

It was almost twelve hours since I'd ridden the shuttle that morning. A different driver took the van from the Allen Pavilion to the main hospital campus at 168th Street. I don't remember if the radio was playing or if other passengers joined me on that ride. I had no idea how I would get home, but the van brought me a few miles closer to where I lived.

The A subway train was running. Although nervous about going underground it seemed like the best option. I saw no buses or taxis on the streets and a seven-mile walk to our apartment would be a long hike on tired feet. I was exhausted and just wanted to get home. It had been a day of intense fear and shock, relieved only by knowing my husband was still in our apartment when the planes hit the World Trade Center. My first words to him were, "Honey, you can be late any time you want." His co-workers on the 31st floor of Tower I made it to safety, except for one person in a wheelchair and the friend who loyally stayed with him to wait for an elevator.

Before going home there was one stop I needed to make: I had to visit my son and see how he was coping. Adam's life had stabilized when he finally began to accept medication and treatment in 1992. Although he was never able to work his ties to the family remained strong. He now lived in a mid-Manhattan high rise near the program he attended.

That morning, when the second plane hit the Twin Towers, John started phoning relatives to let them know he was safe. Our son was among the first people he contacted. After speaking to his father, Adam went to the window in his 22nd floor studio apartment. Beyond the tangle of ramps bringing buses to the Port Authority Bus Terminal he had a clear view of the World Trade Center. He lifted the shade and saw the first building collapse.

When I arrived at his apartment late that evening Adam opened the door to greet me with a hug. The window shade was pulled down; he never raised it again. The room smelled of a day spent chain smoking, and his fingers trembled slightly as he offered me a cigarette. It was not a time to refuse.

The letter

"When will you write me the letter that says I should stop working?" This was a question many employed patients asked when they were about seven months pregnant.

"Will you get paid maternity leave?" I would ask. "I don't want to write a letter saying you have to stop working if it means you will lose your income."

Maternity benefits for working women in the U.S. are among the worst in the world: 178 other countries have national laws that guarantee paid leave for new mothers (and sometimes fathers, too). This is one of the three nations that do not. Patients from much poorer countries, like Mexico or the Dominican Republic, were shocked to learn they would not get a penny from their employer while on leave. Even unpaid time off for the birth of a child is often limited to just four weeks for a normal birth or six for a Cesarean, not enough time to recover from the delivery and adjust to the round-the-clock demands of a newborn. Having to return to work so soon was the number one reason to stop, or never even start, breastfeeding among my patients. This deprived babies of the best type of nutrition and the benefits of fewer illnesses and deaths in the first year of life.

The 1993 federal Family and Medical Leave Act (FMLA) allows up to 12 weeks of unpaid time off work for the birth or adoption of a child. But only employers with 50 or more workers are covered by the law, which omits half of all businesses. To be eligible, a woman must have been at that job for at least a year and worked more than 1,250 hours. To take full advantage of the law, a woman who qualifies must be able to go without a paycheck for three months. I hated filling out all the FMLA paperwork – the form was many pages long – but wanted to help my mothers get as much maternity leave as possible to spend with their new babies.

Several prenatal patients said they were given worse assignments, like climbing ladders or heavy lifting, harassment meant to force them to quit. "My supervisor told me pregnant women are not allowed to work here," reported a woman employed by a big box store.

I made up a form for patients to bring to their employer – asking if they got pregnancy leave, how much time off they could take, and whether or not they would be paid – and often wrote letters to employers requesting light duty, either during pregnancy or after delivery.

Taking a sheet of hospital stationery from my desk to write a letter that might maximize the few benefits she had I told my patient, "I cannot lie." But I could truthfully describe a low postpartum iron count as "severe anemia" even if the new mother suffered no symptoms and was expected to recover quickly. Or I might use the intimidating medical term "diastasis recti" (a common separation of the muscles of a woman's abdomen during and after pregnancy) to convince a boss that a woman should not do heavy lifting. For a patient with varicose veins my letter would request a seated, rather than standing assignment and/or rest periods to elevate her legs.

Advocating for patients is part of a midwife's job – a part I loved to do.

Adele

Adele lived in an Orthodox Jewish community more than an hour away from New York City. Large families were the norm there: I could picture young mothers pushing infants in strollers while a toddler clung to the handlebars on one side and a pre-kindergarten-aged sibling held on to the other.

Barely 24 years old, Adele was having a third child. Her first pregnancy and birth had been normal. The second baby had been breech, coming buttocks first. He weighed only 5 ½ pounds and could have been delivered vaginally by a doctor or midwife with the skills and confidence to do a breech birth, but that hospital's policy forced Adele to have a Cesarean section. Practitioners with experience delivering breeches are getting older and retiring; young doctors and midwives are no longer acquiring those skills. Adele's obstetrician told her that any future births at that hospital would also have to be by Cesarean. Institutional policy did not allow vaginal births after a woman had had one Cesarean. Many hospitals enforce the same rule.

Adele wanted a vaginal birth. She expected to have many more children. Cesareans meant a longer, more painful recovery. How could she care for a big family while convalescing from major abdominal surgery? So in her seventh month she switched her care to New York Presbyterian, a major teaching institution which would not force her into a surgical delivery simply as a matter of policy.

The practicalities of recovering from birth were Adele's concern. I do not know if she was also aware that multiple Cesarean surgeries can lead to potentially life-threatening complications. [See Notes to the Reader.]

Adele was assigned to my care in prenatal clinic. She was healthy, but thin and pale. The old-fashioned blouse and skirt that kept her arms and legs modestly covered made her seem older and dowdy, but in a cotton examining gown she looked like a teenager. Blue veins meandered beneath the skin of her pregnancy-swollen breasts and belly. The baby's size, as estimated by measuring her abdomen, was slightly less than average but appropriate for this petite mother. After I did the vaginal exam, she anxiously asked, "Is there any bleeding?" Her religion forbade physical contact with her husband during bleeding.

"None," I said, showing her the unstained glove with which I had examined her.

Weekly check-ups began in the month before her due date. At each one she requested that I do a vaginal exam to see if her cervix was starting to dilate. Living a long distance from the medical center, she did not want to return home if labor was beginning and risk having to deliver by Cesarean at her local hospital.

"Your cervix is soft but closed," I reported the first three times. "No bleeding." The baby's head was down, in position for a normal birth. At the fourth weekly visit, a few days before the baby was due, her cervix was a fingertip open and there was some blood-tinged mucous on my examining glove. I held up my hand for her to see. This bloody show is a sign that labor has begun, or may soon do so.

"Are you feeling any contractions?" I asked.

"Very mild," said Adele, "More like menstrual cramps."

A woman who has had two other children may have a quick third labor. Or her cervix may open two or three centimeters and remain that way for days before true labor begins. I discussed these possibilities with Adele, admitting "I can't predict which way this labor will go." It was now late morning. We decided that she should take a long walk with her husband, who sat in the waiting room, his black coat and hat incongruous among the big-bellied women in brightly colored summer clothes. Then they could eat lunch: the hospital cafeteria sold some kosher food. After that she would go to Labor and Delivery to be evaluated.

I wrote a referral documenting that she was 1.5 centimeters dilated and her cervix 90 percent effaced (thinned out) at 11:20 a.m. The referral also informed the staff of her desire for a vaginal birth after Cesarean, the fact that the local hospital refused to allow her that choice, and that she lived more than an hour away from our facility. Recent policy changes by the Obstetrics Department prevented midwives from attending the birth of a woman with a previous Cesarean, or one whose labor was being induced or augmented, even though we had safely done so in the past. Adele would be managed only by doctors under these new rules.

"If your cervix has not changed and you are not having contractions when they examine you in the labor room," I said, "they may send you home. But this referral explains your situation."

Adele was nervous and excited as she left, with the referral slip in her purse. "I hope they keep me," she said.

Scheduling a patient to induce (bring on) labor for convenience – usually the doctor's convenience – is something I oppose. Especially in a first-time mother whose cervix is not ready induction often fails, resulting in a Cesarean section that might not have been needed if labor had started on its own. Induction is also much more painful than spontaneous labor. If labor is induced more than a week before the due date there is a danger of delivering the baby prematurely. However, Adele was having her third baby and her cervix already was slightly dilated. She had completed 39 weeks of pregnancy, so the baby was full term. Induction was a safe option under these circumstances, far safer than doing an unnecessary (and unwanted) repeat Cesarean.

A sympathetic doctor admitted my patient that afternoon and induced labor. Before dawn the next morning Adele delivered a healthy 5-pound 15-ounce baby girl vaginally. I was happy for her. That was what Adele wanted. I imagine she has had several more normal births since then.

Sapphire

"The sonogram says my baby is a girl!" Tonia said as she arrived for her 7-month prenatal check-up. "Her name will be Sapphire," she added, stroking her belly. This pregnancy was unplanned, the baby's father out of the picture. In spite of some college education and perfect English, spoken with a sophisticated British accent from her Caribbean country, Tonia struggled to make ends meet. As her pregnancy became more obvious office temp and waitressing jobs were harder to get. The Women, Infants and Children nutrition program that provides healthy food to some 9 million low-income pregnant or nursing women and young children helped stretch her dollars with coupons for milk, eggs, cheese and beans. The baby could get formula from WIC too, but Tonia planned to breastfeed.

Tonia was in her mid-twenties, healthy, a non-smoker, not overweight. She had started prenatal care early and this was her fifth visit with me. Blood tests, other lab work and an ultrasound had all been normal. So were her blood pressure and weight gain today. Her urine showed no sugar or protein. Using a tape measure and carefully feeling her abdomen told me that Sapphire was growing well. I could feel her kick and squirm under my probing fingers.

"She's so active," Tonia said, "a little dancer." Together we listened to the galloping sounds of the fetal heart, 148 beats a minute.

"Isn't it fast?" she said. Many patients asked the same question.

"Fast for an adult but perfect for 7 months. A baby's heart beats about twice as fast as its mother's," I reassured her.

A big part of a midwife's job is encouraging a woman to ask questions and express her fears. You can't answer questions if your attitude prevents patients from asking them in the first place. Stop writing in the chart, stop looking at the computer, turn your full attention to everything a woman says – with words or body language. Listen as if there is all the time in the world for her questions, no matter how many other patients are waiting to be seen. Strive to understand what her question really is about. Thank her for asking questions. Point out that her observations and inquiries help you take better care of her and the baby. Show that she is getting ready to be a good mother by being tuned into and aware of what is going on with her body and her child. Reassure her if a strange or unexpected aspect of pregnancy is normal – but emphasize that she should never hesitate to ask if anything concerns her. Always remain on high alert for the most subtle signs of a problem. And listen to your own intuition when something just does not feel right. Intuition is not a mystical or magical thing. It is the accumulated experience of a lifetime not yet organized into a recognizable pattern.

Tonia's visit ended with my usual reminder to be aware of the baby's movements and warning signs of premature labor, such as bleeding, pain or leaking fluid. We scheduled another appointment in two weeks and she went to the lab to have her blood drawn, routine tests for diabetes and anemia.

Several days later I punched her medical record number into the computer to get the results of those tests. I felt alarmed to see that she had been admitted to the hospital the previous night; labs for diagnosing pre-eclampsia, a serious pregnancy complication, were part of the workup. A pathology report pending on the placenta meant Tonia had already delivered – 12 weeks early. A baby born that prematurely weighs only about two pounds, with immature lungs that would struggle with each breath, and a brain not yet fully developed. My body reacted viscerally with a pounding heartbeat and clenched gut.

Scrolling through the labs with growing anxiety I came to the next item: "autopsy, fetus, results pending." Sapphire had been stillborn.

After clinic I rushed over to the hospital. Tonia was on the postpartum floor where the nurses had given her a private room. Does it seem cruel to put a woman who has lost her baby on a floor where she will hear the rattling bassinets bringing babies to other mothers, listen to newborn cries? Would the quiet of a different floor make her forget her tiny dead daughter? On postpartum units I had observed how whispers about a stillbirth might bring another patient to a bereaved mother's room, somebody who had suffered the same loss with a previous pregnancy and had now delivered a healthy baby. She would comfort the grieving mother in her own way, with her own words, even if they only shared fragments of the same language. Women reaching out this way often brought greater solace than hospital chaplains or social workers trained to do grief counseling.

Tonia sat on the edge of her bed, staring ahead with puffy eyes. "How did this happen?" she said. "I called the ambulance soon after the pain started. When I got here they couldn't find Sapphire's heartbeat."

I knew how to explain the way pre-eclampsia can develop suddenly, without warning symptoms. It causes blood vessels to the placenta to constrict, depriving the baby of oxygen. I knew the right kinds of things to say when a baby is stillborn. I knew the hurtful clichés to avoid. I had attended workshops on perinatal bereavement; I had done this before, too many times. I had even gotten good enough at doing it that I wondered if it meant there was something wrong, very wrong, with me. I did not want to be here with Tonia. I became a midwife because I love the womanly power of birth, not to care for the sick and dying. I wanted to do what normal people do – run away from death and sadness.

But bereaved mothers are the little sisters of my soul. I lost a child, not to the finality of death but to the never-ending shadows of schizophrenia. The pain of hoping, after 30 years, for him to someday be healed still lingers in my heart. I try to use my experience to help others find a path through their grief, a way of salvaging something from my own loss. And deep below all rational thought lurks the fantasy that if I do enough good deeds my son, now approaching middle age with bad teeth and gray hairs in his beard, will magically be restored to health.

Tonia and I spoke for a while, shedding tears together, sharing a small box of flimsy hospital tissues. I kept telling her what a good patient she was, doing everything right, taking good care of herself and Sapphire. Calling the ambulance a few minutes sooner would not have made a difference. It was not her fault that a sudden, unpreventable disease had caused the stillbirth. I could not take away her pain but I wanted to help ease the burden of guilt gripping her heart.

That was the last time I saw Tonia. Because of the stillbirth she was sent to an obstetric specialist in another clinic for follow-up care. Soon afterward I retired, so I never learned if she had another child. But whenever I see or hear of sapphires, I think of her.

Belkis

Belkis had been in labor with her second child for a few hours when I arrived for the overnight shift at 7:30 p.m., fortified by an afternoon nap and strong coffee. She was a prenatal patient of mine; we were glad to be together for the birth. Her pregnancy had been completely normal and her due date was three days ago.

"It started with light cramps after lunch," she said, describing the labor. "Here," she touched the bottom of her abdomen. "At first I didn't pay it no mind. But when Manny came home from work around 4 o'clock," Belkis indicated the large man in the rocking chair, "I told him to take our son to his mother's. I knew it was time, either tonight or en la madrugada," she used the Spanish words meaning in the small hours of the morning or at dawn. When the contractions started coming every five minutes, squeezing strongly, they came to Labor and Delivery. "And I brought my blue card," she said. [See Notes to the Reader.]

The midwife who examined Belkis at 5:20 p.m. found that her cervix was 4 centimeters dilated and 100 percent effaced or thinned out. That is considered early active labor. The baby's position was head first and the fetal heart rate a reassuring 140 beats per minute. The estimated weight of this baby was 8 ½ pounds, slightly heavier than her first child. I measured her abdomen to make my own weight estimate: it was in the same range.

The contractions were now closer together and more intense. Belkis did not want an epidural. She was coping well lying on her side, moaning softly during the pains while her husband rubbed her lower back; between contractions she dozed off. Her behavior was typical of a woman whose cervix was rapidly dilating. A little before 9 p.m. the bag of water around the baby broke, with a gush of clear amniotic fluid.

"Fully dilated," my examination revealed. "You can start pushing whenever you're ready." I removed the wet pad under her hips and replaced it with a dry one. Some women feel an irresistible urge to push as soon as, or even before, the cervix is completely open. Others need to take a break from the intense work of transition, the part of labor when the cervix dilates the final few centimeters, and wait until they feel a strong desire to push.

"I'm ready," said Belkis, grabbing the backs of her thighs and starting to push. Manny supported her head while Darlene, the nurse, adjusted the head of the bed to a higher, more comfortable position.

The mother pushed strongly with each contraction for more than half an hour, but the baby's head did not descend any lower. A second baby is often born by this time, but we couldn't even see the top of its head yet.

"What's taking so long?" Belkis asked. "I didn't have to push so much with my first birth."

"You're doing a good job, but another position might work better to bring the baby's head down," I said. "Can you try getting on your knees? We'll roll the head of the bed all the way up so you can lean your arms and head on it." Belkis was game, and the three of us maneuvered her IV pole, blood pressure cuff and fetal monitor belts as she awkwardly changed from semi-sitting at the foot of the bed to kneeling at its head.

"Uuuh," she grunted with the next contraction, grabbing the headboard and bearing down with the force of gravity assisting her. Suddenly there was the top of the baby's head, peeping out from between her legs.

"Blow, blow, pant like a doggie on a hot day," I ordered, hastily pulling on a pair of sterile gloves.

"Uuuh," Belkis grunted again as the baby's head, shoulders and body went through the several rotations of delivery all at once. It needed no help from me except to catch it (barely).

"It's a girl," I said over the newborn's healthy cries and the father's shocked "Oh my God! Oh my God!"

"Let me see her," said Belkis, looking over her shoulder for the squalling infant on the bed. It took some more maneuvering to get mom and all her equipment turned around again so she could hold the baby. Manny cut the umbilical cord. Both parents were dazed by the speed and ease of the birth once Belkis got off her back and into a vertical position.

But not me. This is an old midwife trick, although in this case it worked even faster than expected. The only obstacle to its use is convincing a mother – who had only seen, heard about or experienced giving birth lying on her back – that a position on hands and knees, standing, squatting or kneeling can be so much better.

It just took minutes for Belkis and Manny to go from dazed to delighted with the speedy delivery and their almost 9-pound baby girl.

"She practically fell out," he kept saying, laughing while he announced the birth to relatives and friends on his cell phone.

Thank you Belkis for being bold enough to try something that was new to you, but that midwives and mothers have been doing forever.

Laboring:

CHAPTER 10

The Bronx revisited, 2012

Gray sky above, sooty gray slush underfoot from yesterday's brief snowfall, on January 22, 2012 I retraced my old path through the Bronx. It has been more than 20 years since I left Lincoln. What would I find?

Exiting the subway at 149th Street and Grand Concourse, I saw that Hostos Community College, just two buildings when I was last here, has expanded to a whole big campus. But the main post office on the Concourse, with its graceful columns and art deco sculptures, was being closed down. One door remained unlocked and I entered the eerily empty interior. Completed in 1937, its walls were decorated with Works Progress Administration-commissioned murals by Ben Shahn and Bernarda Bryson depicting people at work in various occupations. Leaving the building I noticed that across the street from the old post office, like a jackal waiting for a great beast to die, one of those commercial "mail box" stores has been opened.

I walked into Lincoln's main entrance. It was noon on a Sunday, clinics were closed, visiting hours had not yet begun, a quiet time. Hospital police guarding the elevators ignored me. The inside of the elevators were stainless steel, not the cobalt blue I remembered. The fifth floor hallways were freshly painted, beige with pink tones. Posters of mothers and babies decorated the walls. The floors were immaculate, as they were even in the roughest times. The doors that once swung open onto Labor and Delivery had been replaced by electronic security doors. A sign on the wall instructed visitors in both English and Spanish to stand behind the red line, painted on the floor four feet away, and press the buzzer, stating their business to gain entry. The postpartum unit and newborn nursery were also in lockdown. No point trying to get in. I did not belong here anymore.

Outside, 149th Street was lively with discount stores and fast food chains as I walked toward the BX 55 bus stop. The journey up Third Avenue carried me through a landscape much improved from the one I once traveled. New apartment buildings lined the streets; big box and chain supermarkets, pharmacies and clothing stores offered the same products as bargain shopping areas in Manhattan. I was amazed to see a new steel and glass tower rising not far away from the police precinct featured in the 1981 movie "Fort Apache, the Bronx." The octagonal court building with the statue of Justice remained empty, but had been cleaned and its windows bricked over.

A bright mural now decorated the fortress-like Charles R. Drew Middle School. A different crop of storefront churches were scattered along the way and the Futa Islamic Center has been opened to serve the growing population of West African Muslims.

Getting off the bus at East Tremont Avenue I saw a colorful new children's playground on the edge of Crotona Park.

"They refurbished it last summer," a man emptying trash bags told me when I asked him about the park.

The clinic on Arthur Avenue opened in 1939, one of about a dozen identical-looking beige brick Health Department buildings constructed during the WPA era that still serve uninsured people throughout the city. The wrought iron fence around it and bars over the windows were freshly painted pale mint green.

The Bronx is still the poorest urban county in the United States, but to my outsider's eyes it looked greatly improved compared to the streets I traveled thirty years ago. I hope the babies I delivered there in the 1980s can raise their children in a better world.

Epilogue

This book was completed in 2013. Some of the people mentioned in its pages have died. My son, Adam, surviving great adversity, lives independently. We speak every day, visit regularly and love each other very much.

As I started writing these stories, memories and the feelings they evoked came flooding back over the decades. How I missed the intensity of working as a midwife, with fingers, eyes, and ears gathering information about patients as my mind processed it all simultaneously. How I missed the touching, the way my voice rose to a higher pitch when babbling to a baby, became softer when comforting a laboring mother. How I missed the camaraderie of my sister midwives and other co-workers. No longer practicing my profession left me bereft, robbed of my role in the world.

But retirement also freed me to travel and volunteer my skills. After Hurricane Katrina I worked at the Common Ground Clinic in New Orleans. Attending the 2007 meeting of the International Confederation of Midwives in Argentina, I was thrilled to meet colleagues from all over the Americas. We discussed the challenges and opportunities facing our profession in the varied countries of the Western Hemisphere. Health systems in which pregnant women who are insured or wealthy get over-medicalized care and the poor die for lack of the most basic resources tore at the hearts of midwives working at both ends of the spectrum. Seeing women unable to control their reproductive lives with contraception or safe abortions concerned us all. Whether we came from rural Guatemala, urban Brazil, countries along the Andes Mountains, islands in the Caribbean or North America we felt strong bonds in our dedication to the women we serve. We were united in our goal of providing skilled, respectful, midwifery care to women everywhere.

Although I no longer care for pregnant women and deliver their babies, I will always be a midwife.

NOTES TO THE READER

CHAPTER 2

Home births:

In New York State the Prenatal Care and Assistance Program (PCAP) under Medicaid covers the cost of inpatient and outpatient maternity care for women whose income is up to twice the federal poverty level, which was $22,350 for a family of four in 2012. Most other states set the limit lower, at one-third above the federal poverty level. So many reproductive-age women (and their partners) earn low wages or have no jobs that 41 percent of all U.S. births, about 1.7 million babies, were paid for by Medicaid in 2003, the latest year for which there are statistics, according to the March of Dimes.

CHAPTER 6

Housekeepers:

Suctioning the baby's mouth and nose before the body delivers was later eliminated as a routine procedure when amniotic fluid is stained with meconium. Since 2006 the American Academy of Pediatrics and the American Heart Association have advised against this procedure, based on findings that it does not improve newborn outcomes.

CHAPTER 7

Tiffany:

According to a Centers for Disease Control (CDC) fact sheet, "Syphilis is a sexually transmitted disease (STD) caused by the bacterium *Treponema pallidum*.... Many of the signs and symptoms are indistinguishable from those of other diseases," making it hard to diagnose without a blood test. The first stage of syphilis usually starts with a small sore, called a chancre, that is round, hard, painless and very infectious. This will heal without treatment. In the second stage there may be rashes and other symptoms not very different from the flu. These will also go away without treatment. But an untreated infection will silently spread to the brain, nervous system, joints and internal organs. Over time – sometimes decades – it results in paralysis, blindness, dementia and death. A pregnant woman with syphilis can infect her baby, who may be stillborn or have serious mental and physical defects. (http://www.cdc.gov/std/syphilis/stdfact-syphilis.htm) In the late 1980s the numbers of babies born in New York City with congenital (acquired in the womb) syphilis had reached the highest level since penicillin, which can cure this disease, became available in the 1950s.

Chapter 8

Amina:

As of July 2012, guidelines from the National Institutes for Health recommend treating all HIV-positive pregnant women with a regimen of anti-HIV medications to reduce the amount of virus in the mother's body and prevent transmission to the fetus. (http://aidsinfo.nih.gov/contentfiles/lvguidelines/Peri_Recommendations.pdf, accessed May 25, 2013.)

Chapter 9

Damaris:

After delivery of the placenta Pitocin may be used to strengthen the natural contraction of the uterus. Such contraction closes off the vessels that brought blood to the placenta, reducing postpartum bleeding.

Marta:

Rubella is usually a mild viral illness. But if an expectant woman becomes infected, especially in the first three months of gestation (when she may not even realize she is pregnant), she is at high risk of miscarriage or giving birth to a baby with congenital

Laboring:

rubella syndrome. This disease may cause devastating fetal abnormalities of the heart, eyes, liver and spleen as well as mental retardation and deafness. According to the National Network for Immunization Information a 1963-64 rubella outbreak in the United States infected 12 million people and resulted in about 20,000 babies born with permanent disabilities. Since the development of a vaccine in 1969 cases of congenital rubella syndrome have decreased dramatically to fewer than ten annually. (http://www.immunizationinfo.org/vaccines/rubella, accessed Jan. 21, 2013.)

Adele:

A uterus that is repeatedly cut and scarred may cause abnormalities of the placenta in future pregnancies. In placenta previa the placenta is implanted over the cervical opening. As the cervix dilates in labor massive bleeding can kill baby and mother. Immediate surgery is needed to save both lives. Placenta accreta and percreta occur when placental tissue becomes deeply imbedded in the uterine muscle. These placentas cannot be delivered: the entire uterus must be removed, often with severe blood loss. Once extremely rare, these complications are increasingly frequent as Cesarean sections have grown to one-third of all births and vaginal birth after Cesarean or VBAC is not allowed in many institutions. A common complication of surgery of any kind is the formation of scar tissue or adhesions. These can entangle abdominal organs and lead to problems either soon after the operation or decades later.

Belkis:

The "blue card" is a 3-by-5 inch booklet containing all the essential information about a pregnancy. Issued by the Department of Health, it has a line for each prenatal visit and boxes for the various blood tests, labs and sonograms. For many mothers it is a cherished possession, documenting how well they took care of themselves during pregnancy. There is a similar card for babies, in yellow; it shows infant and early childhood growth, development and immunizations. In the days before electronic medical records – and even now when such records are not transferrable between hospitals – the blue card gives vital information. Filling in the blue card at every clinic visit, in addition to the regular chart and billing forms, was extra paperwork. But since it was so meaningful to the mothers, and such an important source of information if there was no chart, the midwives made the effort to write in the patients' week of pregnancy, weight, blood pressure, urine test results and abdomen size at every visit.

Sources

Cochrane Summaries: "Continuous support for women during childbirth," Hodnett ED, Gates S, Hofmeyr G, Sakala C, Published Online: July 15, 2013

Midwifery: Evidence-Based Practice, A Summary of Research on Midwifery Practice in the United States, American College of Nurse-Midwives; revised April 2012

The Atlantic: "The Most Scientific Birth Is Often the Least Technological Birth," Dreger, Alice, March 20, 2012

New York City government HHC website for facts and history about Bellevue and Lincoln.

Book Club Discussion Guide

1. What was your impression of midwives before reading this book?

2. Did that impression change after you read these stories?

3. Do any of the stories remind you of births you experienced or heard about from family or friends?

4. How do the births described in these stories compare to what you have seen on television, in films or on the internet?

About the Author

Ellen Cohen worked as a midwife in New York City hospitals for more than two decades, delivering some 1,400 babies and participating in research that led to the first breakthrough in preventing mother-to-child transmission of the AIDS virus.

Made in the USA
Middletown, DE
26 May 2015